AUTISM SPECTRUM DISORDERS

Selected Titles in ABC-CLIO's
**CONTEMPORARY
WORLD ISSUES**
Series

For a complete list of titles in this series, please visit
www.abc-clio.com.

Books in the Contemporary World Issues series address vital issues in today's society, such as genetic engineering, pollution, and biodiversity. Written by professional writers, scholars, and nonacademic experts, these books are authoritative, clearly written, up-to-date, and objective. They provide a good starting point for research by high school and college students, scholars, and general readers as well as by legislators, businesspeople, activists, and others.

Each book, carefully organized and easy to use, contains an overview of the subject, a detailed chronology, biographical sketches, facts and data and/or documents and other primary-source material, a directory of organizations and agencies, annotated lists of print and nonprint resources, and an index.

Readers of books in the Contemporary World Issues series will find the information they need to have a better understanding of the social, political, environmental, and economic issues facing the world today.

AUTISM SPECTRUM DISORDERS

A Reference Handbook

Raphael Bernier and Jennifer Gerdts

**CONTEMPORARY
WORLD ISSUES**

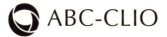 ABC-CLIO

Santa Barbara, California • Denver, Colorado • Oxford, England

Library of Congress Cataloging-in-Publication Data

Bernier, Raphael (Raphael A.)
  Autism spectrum disorders : a reference handbook / Raphael Bernier and Jennifer Gerdts.
       p. ; cm. — (Contemporary world issues)
  Includes bibliographical references and index.
  ISBN 978-1-59884-334-7 (alk. paper) — ISBN 978-1-59884-335-4 (eISBN)   1. Autism spectrum disorders—Handbooks, manuals, etc.
I. Gerdts, Jennifer.   II. Title.   III. Series: Contemporary world issues.
  [DNLM: 1. Child Development Disorders, Pervasive—Resource Guides. WS 39 B528a 2010]
  RC553.A88B47   2010
  618.92'85882—dc22   2010018022

ISBN: 978-1-59884-334-7
EISBN: 978-1-59884-335-4

14   13   12   11   10   1   2   3   4   5

This book is also available on the World Wide Web as an eBook.
Visit www.abc-clio.com for details.

ABC-CLIO, LLC
130 Cremona Drive, P.O. Box 1911
Santa Barbara, California 93116-1911

This book is printed on acid-free paper ∞

Manufactured in the United States of America

To my father who inspired me, my wife who continues to inspire me, and to my daughter who I hope to inspire.
Raphael Bernier

To my husband, Scott, and my parents, Carm, Chris, and Patti. Thanks for your constant and loving support.
Jennifer Gerdts

Contents

Preface

Autism Spectrum Disorder (ASD) is now considered to be the most prevalent of all developmental disorders. The rising prevalence rates (1 in 10,000; 1 in 1,000; 1 in 150; and now 1 in 110), media interest, and celebrity attention in recent years have brought ASD into living rooms across the world. The feeling of personal connection to those diagnosed with ASD is rapidly growing, and whether you know someone personally or are simply interested in learning more, this book can be your formal introduction to ASD.

Autism Spectrum Disorders: A Reference Handbook is designed to provide an overview of ASD for readers interested in learning more about the disorder, exploring the controversies that the field continues to face, understanding the historical and cultural influences of ASD, and becoming aware of the resources and organizations available for the support of individuals, providers, and family members impacted by ASD.

The book begins with a broad overview of what we currently know about ASDs regarding etiology, neuroscience, behavioral presentation, and intervention with a focus on the significant advances of our understanding during the 20th and early 21st centuries. Building upon this foundation, the next chapter of the book addresses the controversies and questions that have impacted the field. These enduring questions are presented within a historical and cultural context intended to provide a broader viewpoint for why these controversies exist and persist. Given the challenges faced by those impacted by ASD and the lack of definitive answers currently available from the scientific community, issues around its cause and most effective treatments are hotly debated. This is evident nowhere more so than the popular media as ASD has increasingly received a tremendous amount of attention in the popular press, television, movies, and even sports over the past decade. As such, in response to scientific findings and celebrity pronouncements, competing theories regarding the etiology of the disorder have risen and taken hold in the ASD community. Given the lack of definitive answers regarding etiology, it follows that there is much controversy around interventions in ASD. The only empirically supported treatments (i.e., behavioral interventions using the principles of Applied Behavioral Analysis) are costly, time intensive, and not effective for every child, while the available alternative treatments lack scientific support and can have dangerous side effects. Through a historical and cultural framework, the origin of these controversial issues and their impact on the field of ASD are discussed.

ASD is, at its core, a disorder of social interaction. Yet social behavior is largely culturally influenced, and what is considered to be socially appropriate in one cultural group may be discouraged in another. In the following chapter, the symptoms of ASD are examined through a cultural lens, and diagnostic rates across ethnicities, nations, and cultural groups are discussed. The historical factors relevant to the field of ASD are clarified in Chapter 4 through an annotated chronology. Beginning in 1911, when the word *autism* was first used by Eugene Bleuler to refer to children with schizophrenia who lost contact with reality, the chronology highlights the important scientific findings, publications, and media events. The historical perspective is continued in the following chapter through a description of the influential people who have played a role in our understanding of ASD in the 20th and 21st centuries. Supporting data and documents relevant to our understanding of ASD, including information about diagnosis, neuroscience, prevalence, and intervention provide a closer look into a variety of components of the ASD scientific field. For example, the diagnostic criteria of the ASDs outlined in the *American Psychiatric Association's Diagnostic and Statistical Manual—Fourth Edition* are reprinted in Chapter 6 to transparently illuminate the diagnostic process. Additionally, examples of behaviorally based intervention tools are described and shown to provide insight into the challenging and important work of behavioral intervention. The book concludes with descriptions of the organizations dedicated to ASDs and a selection of the print and electronic resources available in the field.

There is an ever-increasing amount of information regarding ASD available through the expanding scientific and medical literature, the popular press, and other media outlets. Some of the information is steeped in scientific understanding, while other information lacks credibility and can be harmful to families. The information presented in this handbook is based on the research that we, and others, have conducted at the University of Washington; research from others in the scientific community; and our review of the scientific literature. Our hope is that this handbook provides readers with a comprehensive overview of what is known about ASD with an aim to increase awareness and understanding of the disorder.

Acknowledgments

Providing a broad overview of a disorder as challenging and complex as ASD is a substantial undertaking and would not have been possible without support from the autism community. We are particularly grateful for the encouragement, insight, and comments from our friends and colleagues at the University of Washington Autism Center and the Seattle Children's Autism Center as well as other expert researchers and clinicians around the country. Thanks also to the editors and staff at ABC-CLIO, including Robin Tutt, Jane Messah, and Lauren Thomas who have provided valuable support and guidance along the way during this endeavor. Most importantly, we are grateful to the children and families that we work with everyday who help us to understand the real lives behind the diagnosis and who continually broaden our understanding of the world.

Finally, we would be remiss if we didn't acknowledge the debt of gratitude that we owe to our own families. We can only hope that the many hours we spent behind the computer and in the office away from our families were well worth the final product held in your hands.

1

Background and Overview of Autism Spectrum Disorders (ASDs)

Introduction

Autism Spectrum Disorder (ASD) is a term that has been widely adopted to describe an array of diagnoses, including Autistic Disorder (referred to hereafter as autism), Asperger's Disorder, and Pervasive Developmental Disorder—Not Otherwise Specified (PDD-NOS). Impaired social interactions are a common feature among all three of the diagnoses, and social interactions are considered to be the core area of functioning that is impacted in ASD. Diagnostic criteria for ASDs include impairments in reciprocal social interactions and communication skills as well as the presence of restricted and/or repetitive interests and behaviors. Individuals with ASDs often present with a unique array of symptoms within these domains. ASD is a neurodevelopmental disorder, meaning that it is based in the brain and has an onset in early childhood.

The average age of diagnosis for all ASDs ranges from 3.5 to 5 years of age in the United States (Autism and Developmental Disabilities Monitoring Network 2009). Factors such as lower IQ, being male, and the presence of a regression in skills contribute to a younger age of diagnosis (Shattuck et al. 2009). However, parents of children with ASD often report symptom onset between 12 and 18 months of age (De Giacomo and Fombonne 1998; Rogers and DiLalla 1990), and the early markers of ASD have received recent research attention. In 2007, the Centers for Disease Control and Prevention (CDC, 2007) reported a prevalence rate in the United States of 1 in every 150 children, which is a dramatic increase from reported prevalence rates of approximately 1 in 2,500 reported in decades prior (e.g., Lotter 1966). Two years later, the prevalence rate rose to 1 in every 110 (Autism and Developmental Disabilities Monitoring Network 2009), and 1 in 90 parents reported that their child had a diagnosis on the autism spectrum (Kogan et al. 2009).

Males are more often affected than females, and the sex ratio of males to females with a diagnosis of ASD is approximately 4:1. Most cases of ASD are idiopathic, meaning that they do not have such known causes as brain injury or genetic disease. However, there does appear to be a genetic influence as individuals are at increased risk for developing ASD if they have a positive family history of the disorder. Much research has been conducted examining the brain functioning of individuals with ASD and the neural differences between typically developing individuals and those with ASD.

Many options exist for providing treatment to individuals with ASD. Early intensive behavioral intervention is the recommended treatment approach to address the core symptoms of ASD and is the only treatment that has received positive research support to date. A behavioral intervention approach called Applied Behavior Analysis (ABA) has been studied extensively and has demonstrated promising results in improving outcomes for individuals with ASD.

Brief History of Autism

The term *autism* was first used in the early 20th century by psychiatrist Dr. Eugen Bleuler to describe individuals with schizophrenia who were disconnected from reality (Bleuler 1916). Decades later, Dr. Leo Kanner, a child psychiatrist at Johns Hopkins University, adopted the term to describe a childhood disorder he deemed "early infantile autism" involving challenges in social and language in addition to the presence of repetitive behaviors (Kanner 1943). Dr. Kanner indicated that the group of children he was referring to also had a disconnect from reality as described by Dr. Bleuler, but did not also have schizophrenia. During the same time period in Europe, Dr. Hans Asperger, an Austrian pediatrician practicing in Vienna, described a small group of boys in 1944 with similar challenges in social interaction, but who were not as severely affected as those described by Dr. Kanner (Asperger 1944). He called them "little professors" due to their tendency to discuss subjects in great detail. Dr. Lorna Wing, a psychiatrist in the United Kingdom, later revisited Dr. Asperger's work in the 1980s and encouraged autism experts to view autism as a spectrum of challenges rather than one homogenous disorder. This thinking led to the addition of Asperger's Disorder, among other autism-related diagnoses such as PDD-NOS, to be considered separate diagnoses from autism in 1994 (APA 1994).

Psychoanalytic theory dominated mid-20th-century psychological thought and autism was considered for many years to be rooted in parental rejection of the child. Followers of this "refrigerator mother theory" purported that cold, aloof parenting was the cause of the child's autism. However, many parents of children with autism along with a number of prominent psychiatrists and psychologists rejected this theory. Research in the genetic bases of autism began to take place in the 1970s. In 1977, Dr. Susan Folstein and Sir Michael Rutter published their seminal paper describing identical and fraternal twins with autism and concluded that autism is a genetically based disorder not caused by poor parenting (Folstein and Rutter 1977). This paper was critical in dispelling the refrigerator-mother theory. These findings were replicated and expanded upon in 1995 by a team of researchers led by Dr. Anthony Bailey and provided further support for the role of genetic factors in autism (Bailey et al. 1995).

Dr. Bernard Rimland, an experimental psychologist and father of a child with autism, was an early advocate for a biological explanation of autism (Rimland 1964) and early research in brain development and functioning in children with autism was in part encouraged by Dr. Rimland's writings. Over the years, findings using electrophysiology, neuropsychological testing, postmortem autopsy, and brain imaging have pointed to differences in a range of brain regions in autism including the frontal lobe, the temporal lobe, the limbic system, the cerebellum, and a variety of other brain structures (Akshoomoff, Pierce, and Courchesne 2002; Baron-Cohen 2004; Bauman and Kemper 2005; Hill and Frith 2003). In the years since the early explorations of the neuroscience of autism, many findings have been supported and clarified, highlighting that autism is clearly a disorder that is based in the brain.

Although autism research was conducted and much discussion among clinicians and scientists occurred about autism mid-century, the general public's awareness of autism began to increase in the 1980s. Many have partly attributed this increased awareness to the movie *Rain Man* (1988), which won several Academy Awards, including best picture and best actor for Dustin Hoffman who gave a very accurate portrayal of an adult with autism. Media attention to autism has increased significantly since the early 1990s, leading to even more public awareness and connection with the disorder. Many television reports, documentaries, newspaper articles, and magazine stories about autism have been on the rise in recent years.

Public awareness has been further enhanced by celebrity attention given to the disorder and the influence of several nonprofit organizations such as Autism Speaks who have worked to increase public attention to autism. Such organizations have aided in the provision of increased research and service funding from the government for families of children with autism. For example, Autism Speaks was very influential in passing the Combating Autism Act, signed into law in 2006, which allotted billions of dollars in government expenditures to autism research and clinical services for families.

Domains of Impairment

The core symptom of ASD is considered to be difficulty with reciprocal social interaction, such as limited abilities to develop appropriate peer relationships and decreased shared enjoyment with others. Communication skills are also impacted in ASD. Individuals often struggle to maintain reciprocal conversations and frequently demonstrate unusual speech patterns. The last area of impairment is often the most outwardly striking and involves a pattern of behavior, interests, and activities that are unusually repetitive or restricted in quality. Symptoms in this domain include hand flapping and insistence on maintaining a routine. Each domain will be discussed in detail below.

Although the general areas of challenge are similar across individuals with ASD, a notable reality is that children and individuals with ASD vary significantly in their exact symptom presentation. In fact, experts often conceptualize individuals not as having autism, but rather "autisms" because each child can be so different in his/her presenting strengths and weaknesses. For instance, one child may be particularly good at maintaining consistent eye contact during social interactions, but struggle to maintain age appropriate friendships while another may use appropriate gestures, but have difficulty with direct eye gaze. Taking into account each child's individual symptom profile is important in developing an appropriate case conceptualization as well as focusing on suitable treatment targets.

Reciprocal Social Interaction

Atypicality in the quality of social interactions with others is often considered to be the core symptom of ASD. Difficulties with nonverbal social behaviors, peer relationships, spontaneous seeking to share enjoyment, and social reciprocity are all observed in individuals with ASD. Although verbal exchanges are often a medium of social interaction, much of social intent is actually communicated without language or "nonverbally." Eye contact, gestures, facial expression, and body proxemics are all examples of nonverbal aspects of communication. Individuals with ASD often have difficulty with nonverbal communication in addition to challenges in the social aspects of verbal communication.

Maintaining direct eye contact with others is often challenging in ASD. Some individuals with ASD establish only brief eye contact before looking down. Alternatively, they may look past their social partner's eyes to a point behind them or at another part of their face. Some higher functioning individuals with ASD report that making eye contact is actually acutely uncomfortable for them. Research studies have been conducted in which the direction of eye gaze is followed using eye tracking technology (e.g., Klin et al. 2002; Norbury et al. 2009). These studies suggest that in fact, individuals with ASD tend not to focus on people's faces during social exchanges and instead more often attend to something else of interest in a room such as a light switch on the wall. The pattern of eye gaze is also different in ASD. Whereas typically developing individuals complete a triangle formation with their eye gaze, scanning back and forth between the eyes and down the face, individuals with ASD tend to only briefly look at eyes and more often focus on other aspects of the face during social interactions, such as the mouth (Klin et al. 2002). Much of emotional expression is relayed through the eyes. Therefore, it is theorized that because individuals with ASD do not often focus on the eyes, they are missing cues on emotional expressions in others, making it difficult to accurately gauge others' emotions.

Other aspects of nonverbal communication used to regulate social interaction are also impaired in ASD. For instance, a limited range of facial expressions is often observed in individuals with ASD and/or the facial expression may not match the situation at hand. Some individuals with ASD may laugh at inappropriate times such as when someone gets hurt or may display a flat affect when everyone else is laughing. Body proximity and an altered sense of personal space can be an additional difference observed in ASD, such as standing too close or too far away from a social partner. Gestures like using the hands to indicate the size or shape of something brought up during a conversation or to emphasize a conversational point do not often come naturally to individuals with ASD. In younger children with ASD, gestures such as nodding the head to indicate "yes" or shaking the head to indicate "no" may be absent or rarely used. Some individuals with ASD have difficulty spontaneously sharing their enjoyment of something with others by, for example, holding up and showing the item of interest or commenting on it verbally.

A concept called "joint attention" is also an area of challenge in ASD and delays in joint attention are one of the earliest signs of ASD. Joint attention refers to calling a social partner's attention to an object or action of interest by either pointing and then looking back-and-forth between the object of interest and the social partner *or* using eye gaze alone to bring their attention to the item of interest. Typical infants begin to initiate joint attention at approximately 12 months of age by, for example, using their index finger point out items of interest at a distance, such as airplane in the sky or a train on railroad tracks. Young children with ASD are often significantly delayed in the development of joint attention and frequently need to be taught how to initiate joint attention through intervention.

Peer relationships are often delayed or absent in ASD and parents of children with ASD report that this gap in peer relationships becomes more pronounced as children grow older. Many young children with ASD stay on the perimeter of a group of children who are playing in a playground. They may watch the other children, but do not often join the group on their own initiative or if they do, it is done in an inappropriate way. One boy with autism, Billy, was easily identifiable on the school playground because while the rest of his class would pair up to swing on the swings or gather to play kickball, he often stood at the edge of the playground and lined up sticks in the dirt. Another child with autism, Harlan, told his psychologist that he wanted to make friends at his junior high. His teacher reported that Harlan did appear to want to make friends but he attempted to do so by regaling his peers with facts about whales, one of his very specific interests. Despite looks of annoyance and clear cues that his peers were not interested, he would persist, sometimes following them around the classroom talking to their backs about how blue whales eat. Asking questions about friends and other social partners, taking turns and paying attention to the other person when it is their turn, and offering to share are all important components of social interactions with peers; skills such as these are not intuitive for children with ASD. Often, children with ASD show marked impairments in these subtleties of social interaction.

Parents of children with ASD report that their children often get along better with children who are younger or older than they are, but have specific difficulties with same-aged peers. This can cause particular difficulty in teenage years when peer relationships are such a focus of social development. Parents of teenagers with ASD report that it is the reciprocal nature of friendships that is challenging because many individuals with ASD have difficulty sustaining a back-and-forth exchange. Some individuals may, for instance, remain quiet when someone else brings up a topic of interest or fail to ask them a question about it.

A commonly held misconception about ASD is that all individuals with ASD are not interested in social interaction. Although this is true for some people with ASD, many higher functioning individuals indeed have the motivation to engage in social interactions and have social relationships but do not know how to successfully initiate and maintain these exchanges. Treatment such as social skills groups can be particularly helpful in teaching children with ASD about the details of successful social interaction.

Communication Skills

Communication is also often impacted in ASD and delayed language development, difficulties in initiating and maintaining conversations, presence of repetitive speech, and lack of pretend play skills are common. Many children with ASD are delayed in the development of their first words or phrases. Most typically developing children have single words by 12 months of age and phrase speech that is two to three words in length by 24 months. Many children with ASD develop single words at 24 months or later and phrase speech at 36 months or later. Some children with ASD do not develop spoken language at all in their lifetime, but the percentage of children with ASD who remain nonverbal has decreased in recent years.

For those who develop fluent speech, an often noted challenge is the ability to initiate and maintain age appropriate conversations. In general, individuals tend to be better able to hold conversations about their own topics of interest rather than about someone else's choice of topics. Some individuals with ASD may provide an inappropriate response rather than ask questions about the other person or make an on-topic comment. Comments that are not relevant to the conversation at hand and inflexibility in conversation topics may also be observed. All these factors make the back-and-forth nature of conversation difficult to sustain.

A recent conversation between a fourth-grade student named Cameron with Asperger's Disorder and his clinician went something like this:

> CAMERON: It was awesome with all the dinosaurs but I couldn't see the T-Rex for very long. (Cameron failed to provide any context for the start of the conversation).
>
> CLINICIAN: I'm confused. What dinosaurs? Was this a movie?
>
> CAMERON: The T-Rex, Diplodocus, Raptors, and Brontosaurus, but time was up when I got to the T-Rex. He is big, has a long tail and has little front arms and is a meat-eater. (Cameron failed to acknowledge the clinician's confusion and only responded to the clinician's first question and in a very literal sense—he specified what dinosaurs he saw. He then continued to talk more about the T-Rex, his favorite dinosaur).
>
> CLINICIAN: Oh, were you at . . .
>
> CAMERON: The T stands for Tyrannosaurus. A smaller type of meat eater is the Allosaurus. (Cameron interrupted the clinician in order to finish sharing facts about the T-Rex).
>
> CLINICIAN (RECALLING THE DINOSAURS ON DISPLAY AT THE PACIFIC SCIENCE CENTER):   Oh, you went to the Pacific Science Center . . . (Cameron continued to share facts about dinosaurs with the clinician).

One girl with autism, Julia, responded to a classmate's comment "I had a really great time at soccer practice" by saying, "Yeah." Her classmate made another statement, "I scored two goals and I was so proud of myself!" Again, Julia responded, "Yeah." The classmate further explained, "Those were the first goals I have ever scored and I think I'm going to try really hard to score in our game on Saturday," and Julia replied, "Yeah." Julia learned in her social skills group that she should say something after someone makes a comment about themselves. She memorized the word *yeah* to say in such situations. However, she used *yeah* too many times in this interaction, and the classmate walked away when Julia failed to ask her questions about her soccer practice and did not expand upon her *yeah* statements.

Some unusual aspects of spoken language are also common in ASD. Many individuals with ASD use repetitive language in everyday interactions. For instance, they may repeat phrases that adults say either immediately after they have been said (called echolalia) or some time after they have been said (called delayed echolalia). Another common type of repetitive speech involves repeating lines heard on movies, commercials, and television shows. Although these phrases can be used at random times, they can also be used in a communicative manner. An example would be when a parent asks a child a question (e.g., "Would you like something to eat?") and the child answers the question with a line that is verbatim from a movie, such as "Pokémon's energy is running low and needs replenishment." Although many typically developing children engage in this behavior occasionally, individuals with ASD may regularly use this "stereotyped" speech as part of their everyday language.

The quality of expressive language can also be unusual in terms of the intonation and rhythm of speech. Some individuals with ASD speak in an overly monotone voice (almost sounding robotic) and others have a halting rhythm of speech and take long pauses between words. Parents of higher functioning children with ASD report that their speech can sound as if they are giving a lecture when the children are relaying information about a topic of interest.

Imaginative play skills are also often impacted in ASD. Pretend play is considered to be under the "communication" domain because play skills are often linked to language development. Typically developing children begin to develop pretend play skills before 24 months of age. Early imaginative play skills include pretending to talk on a telephone or play with dolls. Often children with ASD prefer to explore toys for their function rather than engage in interactive pretend play. For example, they may press the buttons on a toy phone or move a doll's arms rather than pretend to talk on the phone or feed the doll with a toy spoon.

Repetitive or Restricted Interests and Behaviors

Many individuals with ASD engage in repetitive patterns of behavior or have restricted interests. Repetitive motor mannerisms, intense interests, and compulsive behaviors represent some of the symptoms within this domain. Although these features may be the most noticeable to the general public, they do not represent the core symptoms of ASD and are not sufficient to diagnose an individual with ASD. Many of these behaviors are also present in individuals with developmental delays without ASD, such as intellectual disability (previously known as *mental retardation*). As children with ASD grow older, the nature of the repetitive/restricted behavior often changes. "Lower order" repetitive behaviors such as hand flapping and lining up toys are more common in younger and more cognitively delayed children with ASD while "higher order" repetitive behaviors often include intense interests and compulsive behaviors and are more common in older and less cognitively impaired children with ASD.

Although restricted and repetitive behaviors can interfere with an individual's functioning, there are also some important benefits to these behavior patterns. For instance, many individuals with ASD are intent on following rules and routine. This can be a positive trait in that they often do not break the rules intentionally and generally attempt to comply with a rule that has been taught. Individuals with ASD often have intense interests in specific topics. Therefore, they often become experts in a given area and have an in-depth knowledge of a particular topic. This can be beneficial in building future careers and hobbies and may be way to encourage learning of other related topics.

Lower Order Repetitive Behavior

Lower order repetitive (also known as stereotyped) behavior includes repetitive motor movements and repeated use of objects in a nonfunctional way. Stereotyped and/or repetitive motor movements (also called motor mannerisms) are common in ASD and involve specific and repetitive ways of moving the body, such as repeated hand flapping, finger flicking, and complex, whole body movements (e.g., rocking back-and-forth while moving the arms). Motor mannerisms may occur more often during stressful situations or periods of excitement than during other neutral times. Repetitive and nonfunctional use of objects is also common, particularly in younger children. Examples include repeatedly waving objects in front of the eyes, lining up toys, repeatedly spinning the wheels of a car, and dropping items from the same distance to watch them fall. These behaviors are called "nonfunctional" because they prevent the use of the objects as they were intended (e.g., focusing on spinning the wheels of a car rather than racing cars along a pretend road). Individuals with ASD are also at greater risk for engaging in self-injurious behaviors such as repeatedly banging their heads or biting their arms.

These types of behaviors (e.g., repeated hand flapping, waving objects in front of eyes, and self-injurious behavior) are often described as self-stimulatory behaviors and are known colloquially as "stimming." The origin of the term came from the philosophy the behaviors persist because they serve to stimulate an individual's brain and sensory experience in some way. There has been much debate over the purpose of these behaviors and another school of thought purports that the behaviors serve actually to calm an individual during times of overstimulation by the external environment. The controversy about the purpose of self-stimulatory behaviors remains unresolved.

Higher Order Repetitive Behavior

Individuals with ASD often have specific interests in topics such as particular video games or certain characters in a television show. Although it is common for typically developing individuals to have interests and preferences, a restricted/repetitive interest differs from typical interests in that conversations often turn to this specific topic, it can be difficult to shift the person's interest to other topics, and this interest can take up the majority of the individual's time for many months and often years. Interrupting an individual when they are talking about this interest or doing something associated with the interest can be challenging. The intense interest may cause significant impairments for the child because it takes away from other functional learning and play in which the child could be engaging. Stereotyped language as described above may also occur in relation to the special interest. In addition to interests that are unusual in their intensity, interests that are unusual in quality may also be observed. Examples include an intense interest in pinecones, clothespins, and lights.

An additional area within the restricted and repetitive pattern of behavior domain is an insistence on sameness. Many individuals with ASD prefer routine and become upset when the routine is altered in some way. Driving the same way to school, keeping a consistent daily schedule, and putting food on the plate in a certain way are examples of these routinized behaviors. Parents may go to great lengths to prepare their children for a change in routine and some choose to adhere strictly to a consistent schedule to help their children's daily functioning. Insistence on sameness can also include rituals that individuals with ASD do in a very particular way or order or insist that others do in a certain way. For instance, they may insist that a social partner say something in an exact way or that they get dressed in a particular order (e.g., first socks, then shirt, then pants). The character portrayed by Dustin Hoffman in the movie *Rain Man* (1988) demonstrated this "insistence on sameness" in his adherence to his television watching and eating schedule. Strict rule adherence is also considered to be part of an insistence on sameness area and is often observed in ASD.

Other Restricted Interests

Although not part of the diagnostic criteria, many individuals with ASD are sensitive to sensory input. Some individuals are quite interested in the sight, feel, sound, taste, or smells of things or people. They may, for example, seek out certain textures or smells, such as repetitively feeling a soft blanket or sniffing people inappropriately. Other sensory experiences can be experienced as quite aversive to individuals with ASD. Repeatedly putting hands over the ears in response to ordinary sounds such as a vacuum cleaner or reacting strongly to certain textures such as tags on clothing are common examples of sensory aversions in ASD.

ASD Diagnosis

Although ASD has neurobiological underpinnings and genetic factors play a role in its development, brain scans and blood tests do not currently exist to diagnose ASD. Instead, diagnosis is based mainly on direct observation of and parent interview about behaviors in the social, communication, and restricted/repetitive behavior domains. Specific symptoms within each domain that are required for a diagnosis on the autism spectrum are described in the *Diagnostic and Statistical Manual for Mental Disorders, Fourth Edition* (*DSM-IV*; APA 1994). Although autism was not listed as a diagnosis in the first edition of the *DSM* (*DSM-I*; APA 1952), the diagnostic term *schizophrenic reaction, childhood type* was listed and was used to capture children presenting with behaviors that resemble what would now be called autism. Autism continued to be considered a part of childhood schizophrenia until the 1980s when it was recognized as its own disorder called "infantile autism" in the publication of the *DSM-III* (APA 1980). Subsequent editions of the *DSM* have further delineated autism diagnoses and currently there are different diagnostic criteria for Autistic Disorder, Asperger's Disorder, and PDD-NOS. A number of well-established tools exist to help make a diagnosis of ASD, including the Autism Diagnostic Observation Schedule (ADOS; Lord et al. 1999) and the Autism Diagnostic Interview-Revised (ADI; Lord, Rutter, and Le Couteur 1994).

The development of the *DSM-V* is underway and significant revisions to the diagnostic process are currently under discussion. Some of the potential modifications include the addition of new subtypes of pervasive developmental disorders (PDDs) and the combination of the social and communication domains of impairment to reflect one focal area of impairment in social communication. The final outcome remains to be determined.

PDDs

ASDs fall under the category of PDDs in the *DSM-IV*. PDDs as a whole are characterized by severe and pervasive impairments in many aspects of an individual's life, including social interactions, communication skills, and presence of stereotyped behaviors. Other diagnoses exist within this category of clinical disorders that are not on the autism spectrum. Clinicians working with individuals with ASD are careful to distinguish these disorders from an ASD. *Clinician* is a general term for people such as psychologists, speech therapists, and treatment providers, who work directly with patients and/or clients. The term is used in clinics and hospitals to distinguish those professionals who work directly with patients and clients from administrative staff.

Autistic Disorder

Autistic Disorder is also known as "autism," "strict autism," or "early infantile autism." The majority of individuals with ASD have the specific diagnosis of autism (~60%) versus Asperger's Disorder (~24%) or PDD-NOS (~16%; Goin-Kochel, Mackintosh, and Myers 2006). Males are more often diagnosed with autism than females and the sex ratio of males to females with autism is approximately 4:1. There have been some reports that females with autism have more severe symptom presentations and decreased cognitive abilities as compared to males.

Autism can be reliably diagnosed at two years of age or older, and diagnosis is generally stable. Like all diagnoses within the category of PDDs, individuals with autism have difficulty in three general domains: social interactions, communication, and restricted/repetitive interests and behaviors. Criteria in the *DSM-IV* specify that a diagnosis of autism is appropriate for individuals who have at least two specific symptoms in the social domain, at least one in the communication domain, and at least one in the restricted/repetitive interests and behaviors domain. In addition to these criteria, six symptoms total across all three domains are required to receive a diagnosis of autism. A portion of these challenges must have had an onset at three years of age or earlier. Like many diagnoses in the *DSM-IV*, they must cause significant impairment in an individual's life and are not better accounted for by other clinical disorders.

Partly due to the symptom count requirements put forth in the *DSM-IV*, children with autism generally experience a greater number of difficulties than those with a diagnosis of Asperger's Disorder or PDD-NOS. Epidemiological studies suggest that approximately 60–70 percent of individuals with autism have co-occurring intellectual disability (Fombonne 2003) and one-third to one-half of those diagnosed with Autistic Disorder have severely impaired language and/or remain nonverbal through adulthood (Howlin et al. 2004). *Intellectual disability* is a diagnostic term used to describe individuals with significantly below-average intellectual abilities that are accompanied by other impairments in daily living behaviors (e.g., self-care, independent living skills, and interpersonal skills). Difficulties must begin early in life and are assessed by an evaluation of cognitive abilities and daily living skills. There are a range of different levels of intellectual disability, from mild to profound. In recent years, diagnoses of intellectual disability have decreased while numbers of autism diagnoses have increased (Croen et al. 2002). Many experts believe that this is due to identifying many children previously labeled with intellectual disability as having autism. In the past, many more children diagnosed with autism had co-occurring intellectual disability and a large percentage were nonverbal for the duration of their lifetime (Rutter, Greenfield, and Lockyer 1967). However, the number of children diagnosed with autism who have intellectual disability and/or do not develop language has decreased substantially in recent years (Croen et al. 2002). This is likely due to a number of factors, including an increased ability to diagnose more subtle and less severe individuals as well as improved interventions that are increasingly available in the community.

Although not a technical *DSM-IV* diagnosis, many clinicians classify individuals with autism according to their cognitive ability level and ability to adapt in their day-to-day lives (called adaptive functioning). Individuals with average cognitive abilities and little impairment in adaptive functioning are often referred to as having "high-functioning autism (HFA)" while those with some form of intellectual disability and challenges in adaptive functioning are referred to as having "low-functioning autism (LFA)." Many children with LFA are also nonverbal. The line between high- and low-functioning autism is often blurred and there is not consensus by professionals as to specific criteria for HFA and LFA.

Individuals with autism experience a greater number of medical conditions as compared to the general population. The exact reasons for this occurrence are unclear at this time. "Associated symptoms" may include sleep disturbances (e.g., difficulty falling and staying asleep), gastrointestinal problems (e.g., constipation and abdominal pain), and neurological problems, including an increased risk for seizures particularly during puberty. They also may have behavioral problems such as extreme temper tantrums, self-injurious behaviors, and aggression. Certain specialists, such as gastroenterologists, sleep specialists, child clinical psychologists, and neurologists are experienced in helping families of individuals with autism to treat these associated symptoms.

Children with autism also often have difficulties with executive functioning skills. Executive functioning refers to a person's ability to engage in independent and self-serving behaviors such as planning and carrying out activities. People with executive functioning impairments may appear to be careless, have difficulty maintaining/shifting attention and staying on task, and struggle to organize themselves and their materials. Executive functioning challenges are not specific to autism. For example, children with Attention Deficit Hyperactivity Disorder (ADHD) also have executive functioning impairments.

Asperger's Disorder
As with the other ASDs, individuals with Asperger's Disorder (also known as Asperger's Syndrome or Asperger Syndrome) have social challenges and restricted/repetitive interests. Specifically, the

DSM-IV requires at least two symptoms in the social domain as well as at least one symptom in the restricted/repetitive interests and behaviors domain. No requirement for challenges in the communication domain is specified. However, individuals with Asperger's Disorder often have difficulty maintaining age appropriate conversations.

Asperger's Disorder differs from autism in a number of ways. One difference is that a diagnosis of Asperger's Disorder rules out individuals with a language delay whereas this is one of the potential symptoms in the communication domain for autism. Additionally, although many children with autism have cognitive challenges, individuals with Asperger's Disorder have average to above-average intelligence as measured by cognitive testing. If an individual did not demonstrate delays in language development and has normal cognitive functioning, but meets full diagnostic criteria for autism (i.e., at least two symptoms in the social domain, at least one in the communication domain, and at least one in the restricted interests/behavior domain, with a total of six symptoms overall across domains), then they would receive a diagnosis of autism instead of Asperger's Disorder. That is, meeting full criteria for Autistic Disorder would override a diagnosis of Asperger's Disorder.

An additional difference is that the observed sex ratio of males to females with Asperger's Disorder is approximately 6:1, which is higher than the 4:1 sex ratio observed in autism. Asperger's Disorder is usually diagnosed later in life as compared to autism. The average age of diagnosis for Asperger's Disorder is 7.2 years of age as compared to 3.1 years of age in individuals with autism (Mandell, Novak, and Zubritsky 2005). This is likely because individuals with Asperger's Disorder do not have a language delay or cognitive impairments. A delay in spoken language or other areas of cognitive development is often one of the earliest indicators of atypical development for parents. Many parents of children with Asperger's Disorder describe their children as being precocious toddlers with strong and early developing verbal skills. Concerns about social development are often not present until children enter into a school setting where direct comparisons with typical social behavior can be made.

Despite these differences, there has been recent controversy about the utility of maintaining a diagnostic boundary between Asperger's Disorder and autism since both diagnoses have core impairments in social interactions. The issue remains unresolved, with some studies finding differences between high-functioning individuals with autism versus Asperger's Disorder and others finding no differences. Future editions of the *DSM* may not distinguish between a diagnosis of autism and Asperger's Disorder.

Strong verbal abilities in individuals with Asperger's Disorder often mask difficulties in other areas of development and professionals (e.g., teachers and clinicians) may mistakenly attribute observed challenges to being stubborn or overly willful. On one hand, individuals with Asperger's Disorder can appear relatively high functioning and can give the impression of being typically developing. However, this can also be a challenge because they may not receive the attention and intervention necessary for improved functioning.

As children with Asperger's Disorder enter teenage years and adulthood, they are at increased risk for developing other kinds of clinical disorders, such as anxiety and depression (Bellini 2004; Russell and Sofronoff 2005). Experts believe this is due to the presence of age appropriate or advanced cognitive skills in individuals with Asperger's Disorder. Strong cognitive skills put individuals with Asperger's Disorder in more complex social environments and cause them to be more self-aware of their difficulties with social interaction. This places them at increased risk for feelings of isolation, sadness, and social anxiety. However, overall, prognosis is better for Asperger's Disorder than for autism and studies suggest that many individuals with Asperger's Disorder are employed and self-sufficient in adulthood.

PDD-NOS

Like many other "not otherwise specified" diagnoses in the *DSM-IV*, a diagnosis of PDD-NOS is appropriate for individuals who display some clinically significant symptoms but do not meet full criteria for any other specific diagnosis in the category of PDDs. PDD-NOS is often described as "atypical autism" because individuals with this diagnosis have autism-like features, but do not meet full criteria for either autism or Asperger's Disorder. As with autism and Asperger's Disorder, severe and pervasive impairment in the development of social interaction is required for a diagnosis of PDD-NOS as is impairment in either verbal or nonverbal communication skills *or* the presence of stereotyped behaviors, interests, and activities.

Individuals may meet criteria for PDD-NOS if, for example, they have a late age of onset of symptoms that precludes them from meeting criteria for autism. They may also present with subthreshold symptoms, meaning that they have some symptoms, but not enough to meet the required symptom counts for either Asperger's Disorder or autism. Additionally, generally children with PDD-NOS have improved language and cognitive skills relative to a child with autism. As a result, PDD-NOS is often considered a milder diagnosis and is associated with improved prognosis as compared to autism.

Course of Onset

For the majority of children with ASD, development of social and communication skills is consistently delayed from an early age and social and communication milestones are slow to progress. In retrospect, most parents of children with ASD report noticing differences in their child's development at 12–18 months of age (De Giacomo and Fombonne 1998; Rogers and DiLalla 1990). In fact, a portion of parents indicate that they were concerned within the first year of life. This type of course of the development of ASD is often referred to "early onset," meaning that differences in development of the domains affected in ASD were noted early in life.

However, a subset of children with ASD develop normally (or near normally) through infancy and then experience a regression in skills at approximately 18–24 months of age. Although a regression in previously acquired skills is associated with other PDDs such as Rett's Disorder and Childhood Disintegrative Disorder, children with ASD who experience regression have very particular losses in the areas of language and social skills. Losses of single words or phrases are specific to ASD and are reported in approximately 20–50 percent of individuals with ASD (Kurita 1985; Luyster et al. 2005).

Until recently, data in the phenomenon of autistic regression had been gathered retrospectively from parents many years after the regression was reported to have occurred. In fact, there was controversy about whether or not autistic regression was a real phenomenon. Home videotape studies confirmed the authenticity of regression in a sample of children with ASD (Werner and Dawson 2005). The sample consisted of children with ASD whose parents reported a regression in social and/or communication skills within the first three years of life, children with ASD whose parents reported that they had impairments before one year of age and did not experience a regression, and typically developing children.

Whenever possible, home videotapes of children's first and second birthday parties were used in an attempt to maintain comparable settings across videotapes and behaviors were coded by raters who did not know their group status. The goal was to capture a child's behavior both before and after the average reported timing of regression occurs. Researchers found that regressed ASD infants used complex babbling and words significantly *more* frequently than both early onset ASD infants and typical infants. Early onset ASD infants pointed significantly less often than regressed and typically developing infants. By the time of the second birthday, the regressed ASD group showed marked delays in language as compared to typical children. Both ASD groups were significantly impaired in social gaze and orienting to name as compared to the typically developing toddlers. This study was important because it provided objective evidence of autistic regression and validated parent reports of a loss in previously acquired skills.

Non-ASD PDDs

There are two other diagnoses called Rett's Disorder and Childhood Disintegrative Disorder that are not part of the autism spectrum, but fall within the category of PDDs. Extra care is given to differentiate Rett's Disorder and Childhood Disintegrative Disorder from ASD. Both Rett's Disorder and Childhood Disintegrative Disorder are associated with significant losses of previously acquired skills and are very rare, with far lower prevalence rates, than ASD.

Rett's Disorder has been reported mostly in females and is characterized by typical development in all areas of functioning, including motor skills, through at the least the first five months of age. Between ages 5 and 48 months, a loss of previously acquired fine motor skills occurs, accompanied by the development of characteristic stereotyped hand movements that involve moving the hands in front of the body as if washing them. Head circumference growth decelerates during this time period and gross motor coordination declines. Significant losses in social interest and language skills also occur and, consequently, children with Rett's Disorder can resemble those with ASD. Rett's Disorder is associated with severe to profound intellectual disability and there is generally little improvement noted after these losses have occurred.

Childhood Disintegrative Disorder generally involves losses in many different areas of functioning following a period of at least 2 years of apparently normal development and must be diagnosed prior to 10 years of age. Generally, children with Childhood Disintegrative Disorder lose language, social skills, adaptive behavior, bowel and/or bladder control, play skills, and motor abilities. However, some children lose just a few of these areas of functioning. Like Rett's Disorder, Childhood Disintegrative Disorder is also associated with severe intellectual disability and can resemble ASD in its social and communication impairments. The sex ratio is equally split between males and females and seizure activity is commonly observed.

Diagnostic Evaluation

A diagnosis of ASD involves direct behavioral observations of the individual as well as an in-depth interview with an individuals' caregiver about presenting skills and challenges. If possible, an individual's teacher may also be contacted to learn more about his/ her functioning in a school environment. This overall diagnostic process is similar for young children as it is for older children, adolescents, and even adults. However, the specific content of the evaluation varies depending on the age and level of functioning of the individual. For instance, an evaluation for ASD for a toddler will generally involve playing with the child with toys while an evaluation for ASD with an adult would be more focused on conversation skills while seated at a table. Given the severity and pervasiveness of challenges associated with ASD, it is unusual for individuals to receive a first-time diagnosis of ASD in adulthood. The majority of individuals who are diagnosed in their lifetime with ASD receive the diagnosis in early childhood. The average age of diagnosis in the United States for all ASDs is currently 5.1 years (Wiggins, Baio, and Rice 2006).

Only certain clinicians are trained to diagnose ASD as it is a complex process involving careful documentation and observation of specific behaviors as well accurate acquisition of developmental history of the presenting concerns. Such clinicians ("diagnosticians") include clinical psychologists, developmental pediatricians, psychiatrists, and some neurologists. Other professionals such as teachers, speech therapists, and occupational therapists who work with children with ASD often refer children to diagnosticians to complete an evaluation.

Diagnostic Tools

A number of gold-standard tools exist to help clinicians diagnose ASD by providing a standardized way to collect and observe relevant information about skills and development. Autism is currently the only childhood mental or developmental disorder for which such well-validated diagnostic tools exist. The ADOS (Lord et al. 1999) is a semistructured and often-used assessment that allows clinicians to obtain information about skills relevant to ASD. It is a play-based measure assessing social and communication skills as well as restricted/repetitive interests and is widely used in both autism research and clinical settings. The ADOS usually lasts 45–60 minutes and consists of 10–14 different play activities designed to elicit social communication. For younger children, parents are often in the room while the clinician is doing the ADOS.

The ADI (Lord, Rutter, and Le Couteur 1994) is also an assessment tool that is helpful in making a diagnosis of ASD. It is a 2–2.5 hour interview that is conducted with a child's primary caregiver. During the ADI, the clinician asks very specific questions about a child's social and language development as well as sensory and repetitive/restricted behaviors and interests. The ADI is more often used in research than clinical settings because it is a lengthy interview. In its stead, clinicians may chose to use a modified intake interview to collect information from parents about developmental history. Questions are generally similar to those on the ADI.

After collecting all relevant information from direct observation of the individual as well as parent interview, clinicians refer to the *DSM-IV* to determine if the child meets criteria for an ASD. The *DSM* is a reference manual that is published by the American Psychiatric Association. It is widely used by clinical providers and provides a description of all of the specific diagnoses of mental disorders and groups these diagnoses by category. A list of symptoms and diagnostic criteria is specified for all of the possible diagnoses. As of 2010, the *DSM* was in its fourth edition. Sections pertaining to ASD will likely be significantly modified in the subsequent edition.

Standardized testing is often conducted during diagnostic evaluations for ASD to determine the individual's level of adaptive and cognitive functioning. Executive functioning, memory, and learning abilities may also be examined. Standardized testing refers to a general category of neuropsychological assessments that have been widely used with individuals of a variety of ages.

The tests are administered using a specific manual and are designed to be given in the same way to every individual who takes the test. This allows the makers of the tests to report "normative scores" (also called "standard scores" or "norms"), which provide the average score for a particular age and/or sex. This allows clinicians to compare an individual's test results to the average results for someone his/her age in order to see how a given person's performance on the test may (or may not) vary from what would be expected. For example, the average score for many cognitive assessments is 100. An earned standard score of 80 on a cognitive assessment generally indicates that the individual is functioning below age expectations as compared to the average person his/her age who takes the test.

Cognitive testing is a type of standardized test that is often given during ASD diagnostic evaluations. This is sometimes referred to as "intelligence testing" and is a general term describing many different assessments that are all designed to provide information about a child's current verbal and nonverbal problem-solving skills. Usually, cognitive testing is done at a table and includes activities such as making patterns with blocks, completing patterns/puzzles, and answering questions about words. Results from a child's cognitive test helps schools and clinicians to better understand what a child's strengths and weaknesses are in terms of learning styles and knowledge-base. Many children with ASDs complete a number of cognitive tests throughout their lifetime either in school or as part of another evaluation. Some of the different cognitive test names include the Wechsler Intelligence Scale for Children, Differential Ability Scales, Stanford-Binet Intelligence Test, and Mullen Scales of Early Learning.

Clinical Vignettes

Autistic Disorder

Connor is a three-year-old boy who was recently diagnosed with autism. His parents were first concerned about his development at 18 months of age because he was not using any words and did not point to make requests or express an interest. He currently has difficulty initiating communication with his parents in any way and it is often difficult for his parents to determine what he wants because he does not gesture or use any word approximations to communicate his needs and wants. Connor appears content to entertain himself and his parents always commented that he was an easy baby because he was so independent.

At preschool, Connor prefers to play alone and does not approach other children to play. When other children approach him, he often walks away or seems to ignore them entirely. Connor often focuses on toys or objects instead of looking his parents in the eyes when playing with them and it is often difficult for his parents to gain his eye contact even when Connor is motivated. His play usually involves lining up cars and other objects in a row and he can engage in this behavior for hours on end. Connor's parents have always commented on his long attention span for this activity and others like it (e.g., taking apart toys and putting them back together). After he lines up toys or takes something apart, he often gets excited and flaps his hands repeatedly near his face.

Asperger's Disorder

Austin is a 12-year-old boy who received a diagnosis of Asperger's Disorder at 5 years of age. His mother was not concerned about his early development because he seemed to meet all of his milestones on time (or early) and was speaking in two- to three-word phrases by 18 months of age. In fact, his mother often called him the "little professor" because he seemed to grasp adult language at a very young age and was interested in seeing how toys went together. Austin has been fascinated by trains since approximately 24 months of age and, as a toddler, he spent hours examining their working parts and memorizing their specific names. Scores on the cognitive testing that was part of his diagnostic evaluation indicated that Austin's verbal skills were in the high range for children his age and his nonverbal skills were above average. Austin could read well before kindergarten and academic performance was not a concern for his mother or the teacher.

Austin began to attend kindergarten at five years old and his mother and teachers noticed at this time that his social interactions with peers were unusual. Although he approached other children to engage with them and was interested in interacting, he often talked only about trains and shared details of his knowledge of trains (e.g., the specific models and makes of various trains and their maximum speed) with other children. The vocabulary words he used were more advanced than other children his age and other children typically had difficulty understanding what he was saying. Holding a back-and-forth conversation with Austin could also be very difficult because he tended to dominate the conversation and rarely responded when others made comments about their interests. Although his conversation skills have improved since this early age, Austin continues to have difficulty maintaining peer relationships and despite reports that he wants to make friends, he does not currently have any close friendships.

PDD-NOS

Charles is an eight-year-old boy who received a diagnosis of PDD-NOS last year. He had numerous prior evaluations and previously received a diagnosis of Attention Deficit Hyperactivity Disorder (ADHD), which was treated unsuccessfully with stimulants, a class of medications that includes Ritalin. His parents reported no concerns about his language development, but did report that Charles has always had difficulty in group settings and often "tries to get out of things" by throwing tantrums. For example, at school, he cries and occasionally becomes aggressive when there is a substitute teacher or a school assembly. Charles has a few friends in the neighborhood, is interested in other children, and can sustain a back-and-forth conversation with his friends. However, his friends usually invite him to play, he rarely initiates interactions with other children, and does better in one-on-one peer interactions than group activities. His eye contact is also inconsistent and he tends to look past his social partners rather than maintain direct eye contact. During the diagnostic evaluation, his tantrums were determined to be aggravated by changes to his day-to-day schedule and to group activities.

Early Identification of ASD

ASD can be reliably diagnosed at 24 months of age. However, parents generally report having been concerned about their child's development much earlier than 24 months, which suggests that there may be red flags of atypical development prior to receiving an actual diagnosis. No well-validated assessment tools exist to diagnose children younger than 24 months, but a number of methods have been used to learn about the earliest signs of ASD. These methods include parent's recollection of their child's behavior prior to diagnosis, analysis of home videos prior to diagnosis, screening large numbers of children with screening checklists and following them prospectively, and identifying infants who are at high-risk for ASD and following them prospectively.

Parent recollections of concerns involving delayed speech and language development are the most commonly reported and are often the primary reason that parents first report concerns to professionals. Analysis of home videotapes of infants and toddlers who later go on to receive an ASD diagnosis reveal atypical patterns of social orienting (e.g., responding to their name and other social sounds), joint attention, imitation, emotion regulation, and reduced use of gestures (Maestro et al. 2001, 2002; Osterling and Dawson 1994; Werner et al. 2000).

In a series of home videotape studies, coders who did not know the infant's future diagnostic status analyzed a number of social, communication, and play behaviors and attempted to classify infants according to diagnostic status. At 12 months of age, coders correctly differentiated infants who later received an ASD diagnosis from typically developing infants in 91 percent of cases using eye gaze, pointing, showing, and responding to name (Osterling and Dawson 1994). At 8–10 months of age, not responding when their name was called by turning and looking toward the parent was the best discriminator between infants with ASD and typically developing infants (Werner et al. 2000). This variable alone correctly classified 77 percent of infants. However, overall, fewer differences in social behavior were apparent at 8–10 months relative to 12 months of age.

The third home videotape study in this series compared 12-month-old infants with either ASD, delayed development unrelated to ASD, or typical development (Osterling, Dawson, and Munson 2002). The inclusion of infants with developmental delays without ASD was important due to the high comorbidity of ASD and intellectual disability as it is essential to distinguish which behaviors are specific to ASD versus general cognitive delays. Orienting to name, looking at people, and the frequency of directed vocalizations correctly identified 87 percent of children with ASD versus those with developmental delays (Osterling, Dawson, and Munson 2002). Therefore, it seems that social behaviors are largely intact in infants with intellectual disability but are impaired in infants with ASD.

The next line of research in identifying early signs of ASD has involved following infants at-risk for ASD until a reliable diagnosis can be made and then comparing their early development with those infants who do not eventually receive an ASD diagnosis. These prospective studies often include either infant siblings of older children with ASDs who are at heightened risk for ASD due to genetic factors or those identified as at-risk by screeners for social communication challenges. Prospective studies have demonstrated that by 12-18 months of age, infants later diagnosed with ASDs show similar difficulties as were noted in the home videotape studies. Impairments in imitation, eye gaze, orienting to name, and early language development (such as social, back-and-forth babbling) have all been found to be predictors of later ASD diagnosis (as reviewed in Zwaigenbaum et al. 2009). Additional early signs have included atypical visual tracking, delayed fine and gross motor skills, delays in play skills, repetitive actions with toys, decreased social smiling and gestures, and slower acquisition of new skills (as reviewed in Zwaigenbaum et al. 2009).

Genetic Factors

Approximately 5–10 percent of individuals diagnosed with ASD have an identifiable disorder with a known inheritance pattern, such as Fragile X syndrome, tuberous sclerosis, and neurofibromatosis. However, for the remaining 90–95 percent of individuals with ASD, there is no known genetic cause or inheritance pattern. Studies examining twins with ASD have found that the likelihood of two identical twins having ASD is 60–95 percent (Bailey et al. 1995; Ritvo et al. 1985) while the likelihood of two fraternal twins or two siblings having ASD is 2.5–8.5 percent (Le Couteur et al. 1996; Ritvo et al. 1989). Since identical twins share 100 percent of their genetic material and fraternal twins/siblings share only 50 percent, the differing concordance rates are often interpreted as evidence that genetic factors play a strong role in the development of ASD. Although the majority of individuals who have a relative with ASD do not develop ASD themselves, they are at heightened risk compared to the general population prevalence rate of 0.9 percent and genetic findings suggest that the risk of developing ASD rises dramatically as the level of shared genes increases.

There has been extensive genetic research conducted with families containing multiple children with ASD (called "multiplex" families). However, the majority of individuals with ASD do not have a significant family history and are the only people in their family with the diagnosis. These "simplex" families represent the most common ASD family type and have received recent genetic research attention. Sebat and colleagues (2007) found that certain genetic abnormalities, called copy number variants—tiny mutations in DNA, were significantly more likely to occur in simplex families than either multiplex or healthy control families. Other studies have found similar results (Bucan et al. 2009; Marshall et al. 2008) and together, these finding suggest that the types of genetic causes of ASD may vary between simplex and multiplex ASD families.

Although many ASD genetic studies have been conducted, there is limited consensus on exact genes that may be implicated in ASD as findings are generally difficult to replicate across studies and research groups. The complexity and variability of the ASD symptom profile presentation may contribute to the difficulty in identifying susceptibility genes. It is likely that many genes, as well as an array of environmental and genetic risk and protective factors, contribute to the social and communication impairments that constitute a diagnosis of ASD. Despite these challenges, genetics is one of the fasting growing research areas in the field of autism and breakthroughs in technology and methodology have become a regular occurrence.

Brain Development

Research studies show that ASD affects a wide range of brain regions. The prefrontal cortex, the medial temporal lobe (particularly the amygdala), and the cerebellum have been shown by multiple research studies to be implicated in ASD. A well-replicated finding in ASD research is that individuals with ASD more often have macrocephaly (i.e., larger brains) as measured by head circumference compared to age-based normative measurements (Courchesne, Carper, and Akshoomoff 2003; Deutsch and Joseph 2003). Head circumference is considered to be a fairly accurate estimation of overall brain size. Although children with ASD do not have larger heads at birth on average, they often experience a rapid growth of head circumference in the first year of life, which then slows after 12 months of age. The relation between head circumference and ASD symptoms is variable and findings across studies are inconsistent. Some studies have found that increased head size in ASD is advantageous and is related to higher IQ (Sacco et al. 2007) and better social skills (Dementieva et al. 2005), while others have reported deleterious relationships, such as an association between macrocephaly and delayed onset of words

(Lainhart et al. 2006) and more impaired social cognition (Sacco et al. 2007). Still other studies have found no direct associations between head circumference and ASD-related symptoms (Deutsch and Joseph 2003).

At two to three years of age, brain imaging studies validate the head circumference research findings and suggest that children with ASD have larger than normal cerebral volume. Technology such as magnetic resonance imaging (MRI) allows scientists to take pictures of the brain and what they have consistently found is that individuals with ASD have an unusually large amygdala, which is associated with emotional functioning and processing (Mosconi et al. 2009).

Cellular abnormalities in the cerebellum have also been noted (Allen and Courchesne 2003;, Courchesne 1997). The cerebellum is involved with complex motor activities, attention, and language. These are all areas of impairment in autism.

In addition to specific brain regions that are shown to be unusual in autism, new technologies have allowed scientists to look at connections between regions of the brain. Researchers have found that there is poor connectivity between different brain regions, particularly between the frontal cortex and other regions, in individuals with autism (Minshew and Williams 2007).

These findings of abnormal brain regions and poor connections between brain regions in autism has led scientists to consider two different theories to account for the social impairments noted in autism. One theory is that specific regions of the brain are impaired—regions of the brain that are involved in social information such as the amygdala and prefrontal cortex. The second theory is that a general impairment in connectivity between brain cells and brain regions results in the impairments in symptoms of autism. According to this theory, it is the connections between brain regions, not focal impairments in those regions themselves, which results in the impairments in autism. Future research using brain imaging techniques hopes to resolve this debate.

Treatments

Despite the strong biological basis of ASD, medical treatments such as medication have not been shown to successfully treat the core symptoms of ASD and behavioral intervention is the only treatment to date with research support demonstrating effectiveness. In particular, ABA has repeatedly been shown to improve ASD symptoms. *ABA* is a general term that encompasses intervention approaches designed to change behavior and is a teaching method of carefully reinforcing certain positive behaviors while decreasing unwanted behaviors.

The first support for using behavioral intervention with young children with autism surfaced in the 1960s and 1970s. Prior to this time, it was assumed that children's symptoms could not improve and that individuals with autism could not gain skills. Individuals with autism, along with others with intellectual disability were often institutionalized in "mental asylums" for the duration of their lifetime where visits from relatives were discouraged. Psychoanalysis was also used as a treatment for autism as it was the main treatment modality recommended for mental disorders during that time period. However, treatment gains were rarely noted in children with autism using psychoanalysis. Pioneering work on behavioral intervention in children with autism was done primarily by O. Ivar Lovaas (Lovaas 1987; Lovaas et al. 1973; Lovaas, Schreibman, and Koegel 1974). Through many years of study, Lovaas found that specifically reinforcing and punishing certain behaviors could shape a child with autism's behavior and produce measurable improvement in the areas targeted in the intervention such as eye contact and development of language. This was a groundbreaking finding given the commonly held assumption of the time that individuals with autism could not learn. Up until approximately the mid-1980s, ABA included physical punishments such as electric shock, spanking, and slapping (Lovaas, Schaeffer, and Simmons 1965). These punishments are no longer recommended in ABA therapy and only reinforcements (not punishments) are used to teach skills.

Social and communication skills are usually the focus of ABA treatment in ASD and skills are generally taught methodically, starting with more foundational skills and moving onto more complex skills. ABA therapy is often done in a home setting by trained therapists but can also be applied in a school setting. Parents can be taught ABA techniques and are often encouraged to use such methods when interacting with their children to maximize treatment responsiveness. A child's ABA therapy program is usually designed by a psychologist or applied behavior analyst and is individualized for each child in order to address and use the child's specific strengths to improve areas of challenge.

The first treatment based on ABA principles was Discrete Trial Training (DTT) and early on the term ABA was used to refer to this specific technique. In DTT a child is reinforced with a reward for each trial to which he or she responds correctly. A trial might be to correctly identify a cup compared to a shoe. Over multiple trials the clinician shapes the child's behavior and through careful monitoring for effectiveness a clinician can determine when it is time to focus on a new skill. This original ABA treatment was conducted in stark rooms for which there was little distraction and the treatment took up to 40 hours each week (Lovaas et al. 1973). Since this original form of ABA treatment, a number of other methods applying these behavioral principles have been established.

Other ABA treatment modalities include Pivotal Response Training (PRT; Schreibman, Kaneko, and Koegel 1991), which was developed by Robert Koegel and Laura Schreibman who worked with Lovaas on his original DTT research. PRT differs from DTT in that it is a more naturalistic intervention based on the principles of ABA. PRT is a type of intervention specific to ASDs that targets two "pivotal" behaviors: motivation and responsiveness to multiple cues. The rationale behind PRT is that by changing these pivotal behaviors, all other areas of functioning are improved as well. PRT works to increase motivation by including components such as child choice, turn-taking, reinforcing attempts and interspersing maintenance tasks.

The Early Start Denver Model is another treatment based on ABA principles. It is an intervention for children with ASD that fuses teaching principles of ABA with a developmental curriculum and relationship-based component. Play is the framework for developing positive social interactions and teaching episodes between the child and the adult. This model was developed by Sally Rogers and Geraldine Dawson, and their collaborators at the University of Washington, the UC Davis M.I.N.D. Institute, and University of Colorado Health Sciences Center (Rogers and Dawson, in press).

Recommendations for ASD intervention (Dawson and Osterling 1997) include beginning treatment as early as possible (between two and four years of age) to capitalize on the brain's plasticity early in life. Treatment should be intensive for maximum effectiveness and 25 hours/week for two years is recommended. Interventions should have a comprehensive curriculum addressing attention, imitation, language, play, and social interaction while being sensitive to normal developmental sequence. Highly supportive teaching strategies should be used that are based on ABA principles and include a protocol for addressing disruptive behaviors that may impede treatment responsiveness. Parent involvement is important as is gradual and careful transition from highly supportive treatment environment to a naturalistic environment. Treatment is best applied by building on an individual's presenting strengths to help compensate for and overcome weaknesses.

Although ABA is the only treatment with research support demonstrating effectiveness in treating ASD symptoms, the number of large-scale, well-conducted studies examining ABA is minimal. This is generally because such studies are very costly and time-intensive. The original study demonstrating effectiveness of ABA in treating ASD was reported by Lovaas (1987) and showed that children receiving early intensive behavioral intervention had significantly higher cognitive scores at treatment termination as compared to a control group and maintained these gains at follow up. Importantly, children in the experimental treatment condition who received ABA were reportedly indistinguishable from typical peers at follow-up. More recent studies with improved methodology are currently being conducted.

In addition to behavioral therapy, individuals with ASD often receive other forms of intervention either in school or in a private setting such as a clinic. Speech therapy is usually recommended for children who receive an ASD diagnosis to help address communication challenges. Speech therapy can focus on improving a child's understanding of other's communication (receptive language), verbal and nonverbal communication (expressive language), and conversation skills. Occupational therapy is also often recommended for children with a diagnosis of an ASD to address sensory difficulties, fine and gross motor deficits, repetitive motor mannerisms, and daily living skills. Given that children with ASDs often have difficulties interacting with other children their age, specific instruction in social skills can often be helpful. Social skills groups (or "Friendship Groups") are available in some places and generally include a small number of children who have a diagnosis of an ASD. Group leaders focus on promoting positive social interactions among group members with hope that the skills learned in the groups will generalize to other settings as well. Topics include starting conversations, maintaining friendships, and improving back-and-forth play. Many children with ASD enjoy these groups and establish friendships in the group setting.

Alternative therapies such as special diets, chelation treatment, and supplemental vitamins are also used by some to treat ASD. However, these have not received research support demonstrating effectiveness and some treatments actually cause harm to the recipients. Decisions for which treatments may be most beneficial for an individual with ASD should always be a joint process between the family and treatment provider.

Children with ASD generally qualify for special education services provided through their school and often have an Individualized Education Program (IEP) to address goals in a school setting. Children with ASDs can range from being in a special education classroom 100 percent of the time, to coming into the special education classroom for one period or one class during the day, to being 100 percent "mainstreamed" in a general education classroom. An increasing number of children with ASD are placed in at least part-time general education settings rather than exclusive special education classrooms. Integrated classrooms also exist, which are classroom environments containing both typically developing children and children with special needs. In these classrooms, typically developing children often serve as models for children with special needs (such as ASD) in learning, for example, social, communication, and academic skills. Speech therapy, occupational therapy, and social skills groups can also be provided in a school setting. The type of services offered at a child's school varies widely among school districts.

Specific treatment aids such as visual supports are particularly helpful for children with ASD. Children with ASD are generally better able to understand their world visually rather than verbally. In order to take advantage of this relative strength, it is often helpful to use visual cues to help children with autism understand verbal information. Techniques such as using small pictures to make requests instead of using words, [Picture Exchange Communication System (PECS)], showing the schedule for the day visually in pictures (called a "visual schedule"), and pairing pictures with verbal information (e.g., "social stories") can be very helpful in maximizing a child's learning and understanding.

PECS is a visual support that is intended to help children communicate through the use of pictures in place of spoken language. PECS was created especially for children with autism who have delayed language development and/or who are nonverbal. In PECS, children approach a communicative partner and give them a picture of a desired item in exchange for that item. Eventually, children can learn to string pictures together to form sentences. PECS can be used to make requests or to comment on the environment. Some parents have expressed concern that their child will become dependent on PECS to communicate rather than developing speech. Research studies have actually found that children develop speech *faster* with PECS than without it (Yoder and Stone 2006).

A visual schedule is a method of providing a schedule for the day or an activity in pictures. Children with ASD often respond better when they can predict the day's events because they are better prepared for transitions, which can be difficult for some children. Encouraging the child to follow along with the schedule can also be helpful in staying on task and transitioning to the next activity.

A social story is a short, developmentally appropriate story that describes a social situation or concept (e.g., a trip to the doctor's office) from beginning to end. It also describes any potential difficulties that may be encountered along the way (e.g., "The shot at the doctor might hurt a little, but my mom will be there and it will be all right"). Social stories are designed to help children with ASD anticipate events and expectations and providing pictures along with the story can also be helpful.

As children gain skills using some of the treatments described above, new treatments are often introduced. For example, young children with a diagnosis of ASD may initially benefit from intensive ABA treatment to learn fundamental skills in a variety of domains, including social, cognitive, and language. Once they have established a firm skill set, children may be ready for group work. Through ABA, one child learned how to successfully maintain eye contact during social interactions, initiate interactive play with the therapist, and make some social comments. However, interactions with peers continued to be a struggle at treatment termination and her treatment providers recommended a social skills group to practice appropriate peer conversation skills, sharing, and playing. Treatment recommendations for older and/or higher functioning children often involves group work instead of or in addition to intensive and individual ABA therapy. Older children, adolescents, and adults with ASD, particularly those who are higher functioning, are at heightened risk for internalizing disorders such as anxiety and depression. Individual therapy using a modified cognitive-behavioral approach can be helpful for addressing these emerging issues later in life (e.g., Wood et al. 2009).

Therapy objectives for adolescents and adults with ASD involve the same general domains as in childhood, including social and communication skills. However, specific therapy goals within those domains often vary. For instance, within the social domain, appropriate play skills with peers may be a focus of treatment in childhood while dating skills and more complex conversation skills may be highlighted in treatment with older adolescents and adults. Daily living skills (e.g., paying bills and house cleaning) and job training are often also targets of intervention with adults with ASD. Identification of community resources and support in helping to coordinate long-term care is critical to providing the best care for adults with ASD. Services provided by some states for individuals with ASD may include provision of supported employment and residential living arrangements. Individuals with ASD who have comorbid intellectual disability are more likely to qualify for such services.

Individuals diagnosed with Asperger's Syndrome often have substantially better outcomes as adults in comparison to individuals diagnosed with Autistic Disorder (Cederlund et al. 2008). This may be accounted for by increased intellectual abilities in this population. Overall, however, the percentage of adults with ASD who are able to live and work independently has increased significantly in recent decades (Howlin et al. 2004).

Conclusion

ASD is a lifelong disorder affecting social interactions and communication skills and is associated with the presence of restricted and repetitive behaviors and interests. Individuals with ASD are as different as individuals without autism, with no individual with ASD having the same pattern of symptoms. There is a range of symptom severity with some individuals having significant impairments, that is, having no speech, limited daily living skills, and profound intellectual disability, and other individuals showing mild impairments, but able to be very successful and live and work independently.

ASD has received much research and media attention in recent years and scientists are making new discoveries in genetics, neuroimaging, early diagnosis, and effective interventions daily. One important advance made within the past decade is that children with ASD can now be diagnosed reliably as early as 24 months of age, although warning signs such as not responding when a child's name is called and inconsistent eye gaze may be present as early as 8 months of age. Much research is being conducted to follow these behaviors from infancy and to develop better diagnostic tools to identify children at younger ages with the goal of starting intervention as early as possible. In some cases, it may be possible to prevent the onset of the disorder with targeted and effective intervention and outcomes of early, intensive behavioral intervention reported to date are promising.

References

Akshoomoff, Natasha, K. Pierce, and Eric Courchesne. 2002. "The Neurobiological Basis of Autism from a Developmental Perspective." *Developmental Psychopathology* 14 (3): 613–34.

Allen, Greg, and Eric Courchesne. 2003. "Differential Effects of Developmental Cerebellar Abnormality on Cognitive and Motor Functions in the Cerebellum: An fMRI Study of Autism." *American Journal of Psychiatry* 160 (2): 262–73.

American Psychiatric Association (APA). 1952. *Diagnostic and Statistical Manual of Mental Disorders, First Edition (DSM-I)*. Washington, D.C.: APA.

American Psychiatric Association (APA). 1980. *Diagnostic and Statistical Manual of Mental Disorders, Third Edition (DSM-III)*. Washington, D.C.: APA.

American Psychiatric Association (APA). 1994. *Diagnostic and Statistical Manual of Mental Disorders, Fourth Edition (DSM-IV)*. Washington, D.C.: APA.

Asperger, Hans. 1944. "Die 'Autistischen Psychopathen' Im Kindesalter." *Archiv Für Psychiatrie und Nervenkrankheitein* 117:76–136.

Autism and Developmental Disabilities Monitoring Network. 2009. "Prevalence of Autism Spectrum Disorders—Autism and Developmental Disabilities Monitoring Network, United States, 2006." *MMWR Surveillance Summary* 58 (10): 1–20.

Bailey, A., A. Le Couteur, I. Gottesman, P. Bolton, E. Simonoff, E. Yuzda, and M. Rutter. 1995. "Autism as a Strongly Genetic Disorder: Evidence from a British Twin Study." *Psychological Medicine* 25 (1): 63–77.

Baron-Cohen, Simon. 2004. "The Cognitive Neuroscience of Autism." *Journal of Neurology and Neurosurgery Psychiatry* 75 (7): 945–48.

Bauman, M. L., and T. L. Kemper. 2005. "Neuroanatomic Observations of the Brain in Autism: A Review and Future Directions." *International Journal of Developmental Neuroscience* 23:183–87.

Bellini, Scott. 2004. "Social Skill Deficits and Anxiety in High-Functioning Adolescents with Autism Spectrum Disorders." *Focus on Autism and Other Developmental Disabilities* 19 (2): 78–86.

Bleuler, Eugen. 1916. *Lehrbuch der Psychiatrie*. Trans. by A. A. Brill as *Textbook of Psychiatry*. New York: Dover, 1951.

Bucan, Maja, Brett S. Abrahams, Kai Wang, Joseph T. Glessner, Edward I. Herman, Lisa I. Sonnenblick, Ana I. Alvarez Retuerto, et al. 2009. "Genome-Wide Analyses of Exonic Copy Number Variants in a Family-Based Study Point to Novel Autism Susceptibility Genes." *PLoS Genet* 5 (6): e1000536.

Cederlund, Mats, Bibbi Hagberg, Eva Billstedt, Christopher Gillberg, and I. Carina Gillberg. 2008. "Asperger Syndrome and Autism: A Comparative Longitudinal Follow-up Study More Than 5 Years after Original Diagnosis." *Journal of Autism and Developmental Disorders* 38 (1): 72–85.

Centers for Disease Control and Prevention. 2007. "Prevalence of Autism Spectrum Disorders—Autism and Developmental Disabilities Monitoring Network, 14 Sites, United States, 2002." *MMWR Surveillance Summaries* 56 (1): 12–28.

Courchesne, Eric. 1997. "Brainstem, Cerebellar and Limbic Neuroanatomical Abnormalities in Autism." *Current Opinion in Neurobiology* 7 (2): 269–78.

Courchesne, Eric, Ruth Carper, and Natasha Akshoomoff. 2003. "Evidence of Brain Overgrowth in the First Year of Life in Autism." *JAMA: Journal of the American Medical Association* 290 (3): 337–44.

Croen, Lisa A., Judith K. Grether, Jenny Hoogstrate, and Steve Selvin. 2002. "The Changing Prevalence of Autism in California." *Journal of Autism and Developmental Disorders* 32 (3): 207–15.

Dawson, Geraldine, and Julie Osterling. 1997. Early Intervention in Autism: Effectiveness and Common Elements of Current Approaches. In *The Effectiveness of Early Intervention: Second Generation Research* (pp. 307–326). edited by Michael Guralnick. Baltimore: Brookes.

De Giacomo, Andrea, and Eric Fombonne. 1998. "Parental Recognition of Developmental Abnormalities in Autism." *European Child and Adolescent Psychiatry* 7 (3): 131–36.

Dementieva, Y. A., D. D. Vance, S. L. Donnelly, L. A. Elston, C. M. Wolpert, S. A. Ravan, G. R. DeLong, R. K. Abramson, H. H. Wright, and M. L. Cuccaro. 2005. "Accelerated Head Growth in Early Development of Individuals with Autism." *Pediatric Neurology* 32 (2): 102–8.

Deutsch, Curtis K., and Robert M. Joseph. 2003. "Brief Report: Cognitive Correlates of Enlarged Head Circumference in Children with Autism." *Journal of Autism and Developmental Disorders* 33 (2): 209–15.

Folstein, Susan, and Michael Rutter. 1977. "Infantile Autism: A Genetic Study of 21 Twin Pairs." *Journal of Child Psychology and Psychiatry* 18 (4): 297–321.

Fombonne, Eric. 2003. "Epidemiological Surveys of Autism and Other Pervasive Developmental Disorders: An Update." *Journal of Autism and Developmental Disorders* 33 (4): 365–82.

Goin-Kochel, Robin P., Virginia H. Mackintosh, and Barbara J. Myers. 2006. "How Many Doctors Does It Take to Make an Autism Spectrum Diagnosis?" *Autism* 10 (5): 439–51.

Hill, E. L., and Uta Frith. 2003. "Understanding Autism: Insights from Mind and Brain." *Philosophical Transactions of the Royal Society B: Biological Sciences* 358:281–89.

Howlin, Patricia, Susan Goode, Jane Hutton, and Michael Rutter. 2004. "Adult Outcome for Children with Autism." *Journal of Child Psychology and Psychiatry* 45 (2): 212–29.

Kanner, Leo. 1943. "Autistic Disturbances of Affective Contact." *Nervous Child* 2:217–50.

Klin, Ami, Warren Jones, Robert Schultz, Fred Volkmar, and Donald Cohen. 2002. "Visual Fixation Patterns during Viewing of Naturalistic Social Situations as Predictors of Social Competence in Individuals with Autism." *Archives of General Psychiatry* 59 (9): 809–16.

Kogan, Michael D., Stephen J. Blumberg, Laura A. Schieve, Coleen A. Boyle, James M. Perrin, Reem M. Ghandour, Gopal K. Singh, et al. 2009. "Prevalence of Parent-Reported Diagnosis of Autism Spectrum Disorder Among Children in the US, 2007." *Pediatrics* 124 (5): 1395–403.

Kurita, Hiroshi. 1985. "Infantile Autism with Speech Loss before the Age of Thirty Months." *Journal of the American Academy of Child Psychiatry* 24 (2): 191–96.

Lainhart, Janet E., Erin D. Bigler, Maureen Bocian, Hilary Coon, Elena Dinh, Geraldine Dawson, Curtis K. Deutsch, et al. 2006. "Head Circumference and Height in Autism: A Study by the Collaborative Program of Excellence in Autism." *American Journal of Medical Genetics A* 140 (21): 2257–74.

Le Couteur, A., A. Bailey, S. Goode, A. Pickles, S. Robertson, I. Gottesman, and M. Rutter. 1996. "A Broader Phenotype of Autism: The Clinical Spectrum in Twins." *Journal of Child Psychology and Psychiatry* 37 (7): 785–801.

Lord, Catherine, Michael Rutter, P. C. DiLavore, and Susan Risi. 1999. *Autism Diagnostic Observation Schedule—WPS (ADOS-WPS).* Los Angeles: Western Psychological Services.

Lord, Catherine, Michael Rutter, and Ann Le Couteur. 1994. "Autism Diagnostic Interview-Revised: A Revised Version of a Diagnostic Interview for Caregivers of Individuals with Possible Pervasive Developmental Disorders." *Journal of Autism and Developmental Disorders* 24 (5): 659–85.

Lotter, Victor. 1966. " Epidemiology of Autistic Conditions in Young Children: I. Prevalence." *Social Psychiatry* 1:124–37.

Lovaas, O. Ivar. 1987. "Behavioral Treatment and Normal Educational and Intellectual Functioning in Young Autistic Children." *Journal of Consulting and Clinical Psychology* 55 (1): 3–9.

Lovaas, O. Ivar, Robert Koegel, James Q. Simmons, and Judith S. Long. 1973. "Some Generalization and Follow-up Measures on Autistic Children in Behavior Therapy." *Journal of Applied Behavior Analysis* 6 (1): 131–66.

Lovaas, O. Ivar, Benson Schaeffer, and James Q. Simmons. 1965. "Building Social Behavior in Autistic Children by Use of Electric Shock." *Journal of Experimental Research in Personality* 1 (2): 99–109.

Lovaas, O. Ivar, Laura Schreibman, and Robert L. Koegel. 1974. "A Behavior Modification Approach to the Treatment of Autistic Children." *Journal of Autism and Childhood Schizophrenia* 4 (2): 111–29.

Luyster, Rhiannon, Jennifer Richler, Susan Risi, Wan-Ling Hsu, Geraldine Dawson, Raphael Bernier, Michelle Dunn, et al. 2005. "Early Regression in Social Communication in Autism Spectrum Disorders: A CPEA Study." *Developmental Neuropsychology* 27 (3): 311–36.

Maestro, Sandra, Filippo Muratoria, Filippo Barbieria, Cristina Casellaa, Valeria Cattaneoa, M. Cristina Cavallaroa, Alessia Cesaria, et al. 2001. "Early Behavioral Development in Autistic Children: The First 2 Years of Life through Home Movies." *Psychopathology* 34 (3): 147–52.

Maestro, Sandra, Filippo Muratori, Maria Cristina Cavallaro, Francesca Pei, Daniel Stern, Bernard Golse, and Francisco Palacio-Espasa. 2002. "Attentional Skills During the First 6 Months of Age in Autism Spectrum Disorder." *Journal of the American Academy of Child and Adolescent Psychiatry* 41 (10): 1239–45.

Mandell, D. S., M. M. Novak, and C. D. Zubritsky. 2005. "Factors Associated with Age of Diagnosis among Children with Autism Spectrum Disorders." *Pediatrics* 116 (6): 1480–6.

Marshall, Christian R., Abdul Noor, John B. Vincent, Anath C. Lionel, Lars Feuk, Jennifer Skaug, Mary Shago, et al. 2008. "Structural Variation of Chromosomes in Autism Spectrum Disorder." *American Journal of Human Genetics* 82 (2): 477–88.

Minshew, Nancy J., and Diane L. Williams. 2007. "The New Neurobiology of Autism: Cortex, Connectivity, and Neuronal Organization." *Archives of Neurology* 64 (7): 945–50.

Mosconi, Matthew W., Heather Cody-Hazlett, Michele D. Poe, Guido Gerig, Rachel Gimpel-Smith, and Joseph Piven. 2009. "Longitudinal Study of Amygdala Volume and Joint Attention in 2- to 4-Year-Old Children with Autism." *Archives of General Psychiatry* 66 (5): 509–16.

Norbury, Courtenay Frazier, Jon Brock, Lucy Cragg, Shiri Einav, Helen Griffiths, and Kate Nation. 2009. "Eye-Movement Patterns Are Associated with Communicative Competence in Autistic Spectrum Disorders." *Journal of Child Psychology and Psychiatry* 50 (7): 834–42.

Osterling, Julie, and Geraldine Dawson. 1994. "Early Recognition of Children with Autism: A Study of First Birthday Home Videotapes." *Journal of Autism and Developmental Disorders* 24 (3): 247–57.

Osterling, Julie A., Geraldine Dawson, and Jeffrey A. Munson. 2002. "Early Recognition of 1-Year-Old Infants with Autism Spectrum Disorder Versus Mental Retardation." *Development and Psychopathology* 14 (2): 239–51.

Rimland, Bernard. 1964. *Infantile Autism*. East Norwalk, CT: Appleton-Century-Crofts.

Ritvo, E. R., B. J. Freeman, A. Mason-Brothers, A. Mo, and A. M. Ritvo. 1985. "Concordance for the Syndrome of Autism in 40 Pairs of Afflicted Twins." *American Journal of Psychiatry* 142 (1): 74–77.

Ritvo, E. R., L. B. Jorde, A. Mason-Brothers, B. J. Freeman, C. Pingree, M. B. Jones, W. M. McMahon, P. B. Petersen, W. R. Jenson, and A. Mo. 1989. "The UCLA—University of Utah Epidemiologic Survey of Autism: Recurrence Risk Estimates and Genetic Counseling." *American Journal of Psychiatry* 146 (8): 1032–36.

Rogers, Sally J., and Geraldine Dawson. 2010. *Early Start Denver Model for Young Children with Autism: Promoting Language, Learning, and Engagement*. New York: Guilford Press.

Rogers, Sally J., and David L. DiLalla. 1990. "Age of Symptom Onset in Young Children with Pervasive Developmental Disorders." *Journal of the American Academy of Child and Adolescent Psychiatry* 29 (6): 863–72.

Russell, Emily, and Kate Sofronoff. 2005. "Anxiety and Social Worries in Children with Asperger Syndrome." *Australian and New Zealand Journal of Psychiatry* 39 (7): 633–38.

Rutter, Michael, D. Greenfield, and L. Lockyer. 1967. "A Five to Fifteen Year Follow-up Study of Infantile Psychosis. II. Social and Behavioural Outcome." *British Journal of Psychiatry* 113:1183–99.

Sacco, Roberto, Roberto Militernib, Alessandro Frollib, Carmela Bravaccioc, Antonella Grittib, Maurizio Eliad, Paolo Curatoloe, et al. 2007. "Clinical, Morphological, and Biochemical Correlates of Head Circumference in Autism." *Biological Psychiatry* 62 (9): 1038–47.

Schreibman, Laura, Wendy M. Kaneko, and Robert L. Koegel. 1991. "Positive Affect of Parents of Autistic Children: A Comparison across Two Teaching Techniques." *Behavior Therapy* 22 (4): 479–90.

Sebat, Jonathan, B. Lakshmi, Dheeraj Malhotra, Jennifer Troge, Christa Lese-Martin, Tom Walsh, Boris Yamrom, et al. 2007. "Strong Association of De Novo Copy Number Mutations with Autism." *Science* 316 (5823): 445–49.

Shattuck, Paul T., Maureen Durkin, Matthew Maenner, Craig New-schaffer, David S. Mandell, Lisa Wiggins, Li-Ching Lee, et al. 2009. "Timing of Identification among Children with an Autism Spectrum Disorder: Findings from a Population-Based Surveillance Study." *Journal of the American Academy of Child and Adolescent Psychiatry* 48 (5): 474–83.

Werner, Emily, and Geraldine Dawson. 2005. "Validation of the Phenomenon of Autistic Regression Using Home Videotapes." *Archives of General Psychiatry* 62 (8): 889–95.

Werner, Emily, Geraldine Dawson, Julie Osterling, and Nuhad Dinno. 2000. "Brief Report: Recognition of Autism Spectrum Disorder before One Year of Age: A Retrospective Study Based on Home Videotapes." *Journal of Autism and Developmental Disorders* 30 (2): 157–62.

Wiggins, Lisa D., Jon Baio, and Catherine Rice. 2006. "Examination of the Time between First Evaluation and First Autism Spectrum Diagnosis in a Population-Based Sample." *Journal of Developmental and Behavioral Pediatrics* 27 (2): S79–S87.

Wood, Jeffrey J., Amy Drahota, Karen Sze, Kim Har, Angela Chiu, and David A. Langer. 2009. "Cognitive Behavioral Therapy for Anxiety in Children with Autism Spectrum Disorders: A Randomized, Controlled Trial." *Journal of Child Psychology and Psychiatry* 50 (3): 224–34.

Yoder, Paul, and Wendy L. Stone. 2006. "A Randomized Comparison of the Effect of Two Prelinguistic Communication Interventions on the Acquisition of Spoken Communication in Preschoolers with ASD." *Journal of Speech, Language, and Hearing Research* 49 (4): 698–711.

Zwaigenbaum, Lonnie, Susan Bryson, Catherine Lord, Sally Rogers, Alice Carter, Leslie Carver, Kasia Chawarska, et al. 2009. "Clinical Assessment and Management of Toddlers with Suspected Autism Spectrum Disorder: Insights from Studies of High-Risk Infants." *Pediatrics* 123 (5): 1383–91.

2

Controversies, Problems, and Solutions in the Field of ASD

"Time to get on the bus. Time to get on the bus," six-year-old Jimmy repeated while standing up from his seat, clearly agitated. He was seated at a knee-high table across from the psychologist who was working with Jimmy during the diagnostic evaluation. Jimmy's mother, seated at his side, helped redirect him to his chair and glanced over at the psychologist and explained, "That means he does not want to do this task anymore. He uses that phrase when he wants to leave, regardless of whether he is getting on the bus for school or just wanting to leave the room." The psychologist nodded and switched activities, "Jimmy, let's play with these toys, then." The diagnostician placed the toys in front of Jimmy noting that the young boy did not respond to his statement nor was he making eye contact with him or his mother. Instead Jimmy was focused on the table leg closest to him and was peering intently at the edges of the metallic, cylindrical table leg. "Let's play with these toys," the psychologist instructed again in an attempt to get Jimmy's attention. On the fourth prompt, Jimmy looked up, fleetingly made eye contact, and then exclaimed, "Oh, Hermione from Harry Potter," when he caught sight of the action figure on the table. The psychologist noted that Jimmy made this statement with a perfectly imitated British accent. Jimmy grabbed the Hermione action figure and toy dinosaur from the table and turned away from his mother and the psychologist. Balancing the toys on the back of his chair, he murmured under his breath, again in a British accent, "Hermione is friends with Harry Potter. Harry Potter is a sorcerer."

After several unsuccessful attempts to draw Jimmy back to the table and into an interaction, the psychologist turned his attention

43

to asking Jimmy's mother about the boy's early development. She highlighted reduced interest in interacting with family members and other children, delays in language and use of repetitive phrases, intense interests in specific areas, such as Harry Potter, and regular repetitive motor mannerisms. After reviewing his early development Jimmy's mother asked, "So what caused this? Was it something I did wrong or is there something he was exposed to after he was born that caused his behaviors?" The psychologist shook his head and said, "Certainly not something you did, but you're not the first parent to ask this question. Many scientists have asked, and are still asking, similar questions about what causes autism." Jimmy's mother quickly followed up, "Well, then if we don't know what causes it, can I do anything to help Jimmy?" The psychologist smiled warmly, "Again, a tough question and one not without controversy. The good news is that there are many effective interventions available to help Jimmy. However, there are also plenty of interventions that we don't know enough about their effectiveness and some that have been shown to be ineffective."

Interactions and conversations like this happen throughout the country on a daily basis as physicians and psychologists work with families to identify and diagnose autism and provide treatment options. The questions that parents pose to clinicians and scientists are poignant in that the lack of definitive answers can have a huge impact on a family's experience, development and growth. Unfortunately, science does not move forward as quickly as families want or need.

The number of children receiving a diagnosis of autism and requiring intervention services rises daily. However, there are limited diagnostic and evaluation centers staffed by professionals with expertise in autism, which results in long wait lists for families. A formal diagnosis is important in defining appropriate treatments and a requirement in many states and school systems to receive treatment. We know that the earlier intervention starts, the better the outcome for most children because of the ability for treatment to positively impact the altered trajectory of development in autism. Each month that a family sits on a wait list without receiving a diagnosis, is one more month that the child is not receiving intervention. The problems of understanding the causes of autism, why there is a rise in the prevalence rates, and how we can treat it are paramount to helping families that are working to provide the best possible futures for their children. Scientists, clinicians, and parents have worked to answer these imperative questions and, as in all areas of science and medicine, false leads have been pursued and championed and some conflict has resulted. However, despite these controversies, clear advances have also been made in the field of autism. There is currently great interest and focus in the field of autism and new advances in our understanding of autism are being made every day. The controversies that have plagued the field have been part of the growing pains of a young subject of scientific inquiry.

Controversies Surrounding the Causes of Autism

Our understanding of the etiology of autism has come a long way since Leo Kanner's first description of the disorder in 1943. However, further progress still needs to be made. In the mid-1940s, psychoanalytic thought predominated psychological theory, an awareness of childhood mental illness was just beginning to take shape, treatment for most mental illness was limited and confined to residential placement, and it would not be another decade before Watson and Crick could announce that they discovered the secret of life in the double helix. In the century since the term *autism* was first used to refer to the withdrawal from the outside world shown by individuals diagnosed with schizophrenia, significant advances in science, medicine, and understanding of development have profoundly impacted the furthering of understanding the origins of autism. The development of technologies to image the brain, to scan the entirety of the genome, and to classify behaviors has provided the means for scientists to disprove or support theories and move our understanding of autism forward. Certainly the process has not been easy for scientists and parents alike and controversies have dotted the landscape of the study of the causes of autism.

The Refrigerator Mother Theory and the Birth of the Genetics of Autism

The first predominant theory regarding the cause of autism was that autism resulted from pathological parenting. Termed the "refrigerator mother theory," this theory proposed that the mothers of children with autism respond abnormally and psychologically harmfully to normal childhood behaviors due to their psychological coldness and aloofness—their refrigerator personalities. According to Bruno Bettelheim, the champion of this theory, it is the mother's coldness that ultimately results in the child turning inward and retreating into autism.

In order to understand how this theory originated, it is important to understand the prevailing atmosphere of psychological understanding of the middle of the 20th century. While this theory may seem out of place in the early 21st century given our current understanding of mental illness, child development, biology, and genetics, during the time of its development, it followed directly from the established psychological perspectives.

In the middle of the 20th century, psychoanalytic theory was the prominent perspective on the development of mental illness. Sigmund Freud, considered to be the founder of the field of psychology, developed psychoanalytic theory in the late 19th and early 20th centuries. Followers of Freud have built upon and expanded this school of thought and aspects of his psychological theories continue on today. Although there are a number of schools of thought and divisions within the field, psychoanalytic theory generally purports that mental illness results from unconscious conflicts that follow from early childhood experiences, predominantly relationships with parents. Concepts that are common in today's language and culture are the result of many of the writings from psychoanalytic thought, such as the terms *anal retentive* and *oral fixation*, and the concepts of denial, the unconscious, and dream analysis. Followers of psychoanalytic thought focus on a child's early relationships to explain disordered or abnormal behavior as these early relationships are considered to be the most important features of a child's early social experiences. Extending this viewpoint, if a parent, particularly the mother, is considered to be the most important aspect of a child's early development and unconscious conflicts resulting from early development are believed to be the root cause of mental illness, then clearly parents could be considered the causal factor in the development of mental disorders.

Psychologists and physicians of the early 20th century working with individuals for whom there was no identifiable cause of their disorder ascribed to the predominantly held notion that parents played a causal role in the development of their mental difficulties. Bruno Bettelheim, a professor of psychology at the University of Chicago and director of a school for children with emotional disturbances, developed his refrigerator mother theory on the cause of autism within this framework of psychoanalytic thought. But, it was not based on his clinical observations alone that he considered the parents' personalities to be a contributing factor. This notion of "coldness" in parents of children with autism was actually described in Leo Kanner's first account of autism.

In 1943, in a paper titled, "Autistic Disturbances of Affective Content," Johns Hopkins professor, Leo Kanner, reported on 11 children with "an inability to relate themselves in the ordinary way to people and situations" (p. 242). In this seminal paper outlining the behaviors of these children with "early infantile autism," Kanner mentioned the traits of the parents as well. In the conclusion of the paper, he noted, "one other fact stands out prominently. In the whole group, there are very few really warmhearted fathers and mothers" (p. 250). Despite these observations, Kanner concluded that parent personalities did not cause autism and ended his groundbreaking paper with, "we must, then, assume that these children have come into the world with innate inability to form the usual, biologically provided affective contact with people" (p. 250).

Kanner highlighted that his conclusion was that autism was an innate disorder, not caused by parents. In fact, the lack of warmth Kanner reported observing in the parents of the children with autism in his sample could just as easily have resulted from having a child with autism. That is, instead of concluding that parent personality resulted in a child with autism, it could have been theorized that having a child with a disability results in parental stress and emotional distance. However, the prevailing current of psychoanalytic theory held stronger sway.

With the convergence of the prevailing viewpoint of psychoanalytic theory and the anecdotal reports of parent personalities in the 11 children with autism in Kanner's 1943 report, Bruno Bettelheim posited the refrigerator mother theory of autism. Basing his theory in psychoanalytic thought, Dr. Bettelheim contrasted the behavior of parents with autism to parents of typically developing children. Specifically, he stated that in normal development, as children progress and interact with the world around them, at times they withdraw in response to frustrations or obstacles along the way. Typically, parents respond to the child's withdrawal to the threats of the world with increased warmth, cuddling, and care. The child experiences this care and reassurance and the child reengages with the world around him or her.

In contrast, according to the refrigerator mother theory, parents of children with autism, because of their psychological pathology of coldness and aloofness, respond to normal childhood withdrawal with rejection and negativity. In turn, the child perceives this as hostility and threat, which intensifies his or her withdrawal. The cycle continues to repeat until the child is lost to autism. In his 1967 book, *The Empty Fortress: Infantile Autism and the Birth of the Self*, Dr. Bettelheim summarized his theory: "In those children destined to become autistic their oversensitivity to the mother's emotions may be such that they try, in defense, to blot out what is too destructive an experience for them. Little is known about the relation between the development of the child's feelings and his cognition. But to blot out emotional experience probably impedes the development of cognition, and it may be that the two reinforce each other till autism results" (p. 398).

As one can imagine, the impact of this theory was felt throughout the parent community. Guilt, shame, and pain accompanied the already challenging day to day experience for parents trying to raise a child with a significant disability. Unfortunately, at the time, there was little more that science could provide in the way of insight into the cause of autism. However, there were advocates for the theory that autism's cause was rooted in neurological impairment and biology, not pathological parenting.

Dr. Bernard Rimland, an experimental psychologist and the parent of a child with autism, joined forces with Dr. Ruth Sullivan and other parents and founded what is now called the Autism Society of America. Through the development of a parent-run organization focusing on advocacy, research, and support, the notion that autism was caused by cold, aloof parenting could be examined and the veracity of its statements tested.

Over the years many arguments and questions were posed to counter the refrigerator mother theory. One primary argument against the refrigerator mother theory was that not all parents of children with autism, even children that fit Kanner's classical, prototypical examples, are cold or aloof as Kanner mentioned. In fact, most are not. The second argument consistently noted was that many parents that fit Kanner's description of cold and aloof do not have children with autism. A third argument was that many siblings of children with autism do not themselves have autism. How could this theory account for these three inconsistencies? If autism is indeed caused by refrigerator mothers, we would expect that all (or at least most) parents of autism would be cold and aloof, that all (or at least most) children of aloof parents would have autism, and that all (or at least most) siblings of autism would also have autism. These logical extensions of the theory were not observed.

Other counterarguments were presented as well including the observation that many children with autism demonstrate atypical developmental trajectories from birth, far too early for parenting to have an effect and that some autistic symptomology is similar to that of symptoms shown following brain damage. Many of these arguments were presented in Dr. Rimland's 1964 review of what was known about autism. His book, *Infantile Autism,* highlighted the rationale for a biological basis of the disorder and did much to allay the guilt and shame of parents and drive the scientific community to explore biological causes of autism (Rimland 1964). In total, over the years, a large number of counterarguments were presented to refute the refrigerator mother theory, but the strong influence of psychoanalytic theory coupled with a lack of a specific, definitive alternative causal mechanism carried the pathological parenting theory forward for many years.

Finally, in 1977, with a landmark publication of a twin study conducted in England, the refrigerator mother theory was finally left out in the cold. Dr. Susan Folstein, a child psychiatrist from the United States, and Sir Michael Rutter, a British child psychiatrist considered by many to be the father of child psychology, reported their findings from 21 twin pairs and concluded that autism is predominantly a genetic disorder (Folstein and Rutter 1977).

Drs. Folstein and Rutter used what we know about twins to answer questions about the role genetics might play in the disorder. Monozygotic twins, or identical twins, share nearly identical genetic structure while dizygotic, or fraternal twins, share approximately 50 percent of their genes—the same as nontwin siblings. By comparing the concordance rate of autism in monozygotic twins, that is the rate in which both twins have autism, to the concordance rate of autism in dizygotic twins, the contribution of genetics or environment to the disorder can be estimated. If autism is caused by environmental factors, such as cold parenting, it would be expected that both types of twins, monozygotic and dizygotic, would have the same concordance rate. This is because, presumably, the environment would have a similar impact on both same-aged children raised in the same environment. In contrast, if autism is caused by genetic factors, then it would be expected that despite growing up in a similar environment the monozygotic twins would have a higher concordance rate because they share the same genes.

In this study, Drs. Folstein and Rutter cast a wide net to identify same sex twins with autism. Same sex twins were sought because the rate of autism varies by gender. Boys are three or four times more likely to have autism than girls. As a result, female monozygotic twins, male-female dizygotic twins (and same sex dizygotic twins), and male monozygotic twins would all naturally have different rates of autism due to gender differences and not simply genetic differences. Additionally, a large enough sample of children observed by the scientists to confirm a diagnosis of autism was needed to draw definitive conclusions.

After carefully identifying, recruiting, and evaluating as many twin pairs as possible for which at least one child had a diagnosis of autism, Drs. Folstein and Rutter examined the concordance rate. They found that not one of the dizygotic (fraternal) twin pairs were concordant for autism. When one of the twin pairs had autism, his sibling did not. However, 4 of the 11 monozygotic (identical) twin pairs were concordant for autism; 36 percent of the twins both had autism. Statistically speaking, the likelihood that chance alone could explain this pattern of differential concordance rates in identical versus fraternal twins is less than 5 percent.

This finding provided definitive evidence against the refrigerator mother theory and suggested a clear alternative to the cause of autism—genetics. In the intervening years between Kanner's first report of autism and subsequent examination of the disorder by other scientists, changes were taking place in the field of biology that allowed for more advanced scientific questions to be asked and answered. James Watson and Francis Crick, the Nobel Prize–winning biologists, identified the structure of the double helix thereby providing a molecular basis for genetic transmission of disease and mental illness. Pictures of the brain were made available through computerized tomography providing insight into brain structure and function. Advances were also made in the understanding of other mental illnesses. For example, researchers studying schizophrenia maintained the position that genetics are a primary causal mechanism. Given these advances in science, alternatives to pathological parenting could then be provided to account for behavioral disorders for which no known medical cause could be identified. Autism was the perfect example of a disorder for which no known specific medical cause could be identified. Drs. Folstein and Rutter concluded on the basis of their findings in twins that the difference in concordance rates "clearly points strongly to the importance of genetic factors in the aetiology of autism" (Folstein and Rutter 1977, p. 307). A new era in understanding the causes of autism was born.

In the years following the Folstein and Rutter paper, scientists studying the causes of autism examined all aspects of autism including the effectiveness of different treatment options; early development and the behaviors and symptoms associated with autism, such as imitation and repetitive behaviors; brain structure and function through autopsy and technologies, such as electroencephalography (EEG), positron emission tomography (PET), magnetic resonance imaging (MRI); functional magnetic resonance imaging (fMRI); and genetics through expanded twin studies, genome wide linkage studies, and candidate gene studies. Parents became increasingly more involved in autism research, which helped speed advances in understanding through active family participation in large studies and a louder voice in lobbying for federal research dollars. In the late 1990s and early 2000s, other parent groups, such as the National Alliance for Autism Research, Cure Autism Now, and Autism Speaks, joined the ranks of the existing Autism Society of America and worked to provide funding for autism research. Although the time when parents were sideline observers in autism research and held to blame for the cause of disorder had come to end, the controversies in understanding the causes of autism did not end there. Further, the controversies regarding the origins of autism were compounded by reports of an increase in the prevalence of the disorder.

"The Autism Epidemic"

Increasing rates of autism have been reported in the media and the term epidemic has been included in more than one article headline: "Is the Autism Epidemic a Myth?" (Wallis 2007); "Scientists Challenge Claims of Steep Rise in Autism" (Derbyshire and Brahic 2002); and "Autism Epidemic Being Ignored" (Taylor 2007). Those in the public eye have reported similarly. "We have an autism epidemic on our hands," Dan Burton, Representative of Indiana, declared in 2001 (Lilienfeld and Arkowitz 2007, p. 58).

The spark in the autism epidemic issue was a 1999 report generated by California's Department of Developmental Services that reported a 273 percent increase in the number of children with an ASD entering the regional treatment center system over the course of 11 years (Department of Developmental Services 1999). Since the 1999 report, there have been a number of scientifically conducted epidemiological studies assessing the prevalence and incidence rates for autism. (The prevalence is the number of individuals with a given disorder in a population at a given time, while the incidence rate indicates the number of new cases in a given time period.) These studies indicate that the current estimate for the prevalence of autism is approximately 1 in 110 children. This number is a vast increase over the estimates that existed prior to the 1990s. Previous estimates were approximately 1 in 2,500.

There are a number of complicating factors that make it impossible to compare the current prevalence estimate of 1 in 110 children with a diagnosis to the previous 1 in 2,500 estimate that existed for many years. These include changes in diagnostic criteria, increased awareness and greater access to services, financial incentives, and changes in epidemiological methodology and reporting procedures.

Firstly, the diagnostic criteria for autism have changed considerably in the past 20 years. The *Diagnostic and Statistical Manual of Mental Disorders* (*DSM*) is the reference book for psychiatry and psychology. It is currently undergoing its fifth revision. With each revision, diagnostic boundaries are modified and criteria adjusted to reflect new scientific research (and cultural influences). As the landscape in autism is consistently shifting, so is the field of psychiatry and psychology in general and this is reflected in the *DSM*. For example, in the first edition of the *DSM*, homosexuality was listed as a mental disorder. Thankfully, advances in research and cultural awareness were incorporated in the *DSM* revision process and homosexuality was removed from the manual in 1974. Substantial changes were made to the diagnostic criteria for autism through the *DSM* revision process, including the addition of two additional subtypes of Pervasive Developmental Disorders: Asperger's Disorder and Pervasive Developmental Disorder— Not Otherwise Specified (PPD-NOS). The inclusion of these additional subtypes involved the loosening of diagnostic criteria. That meant that more people could meet diagnostic criteria for an ASD when these changes took place in 1987 with the development of the *DSM-III-R* and again in 1994 with the *DSM-IV*. Previous prevalence rates, therefore, considered only what would now be classified as Autistic Disorder, while the current 1 in 110 prevalence rates include all three diagnoses in the autism spectrum. The author of the 2007 *Unstrange Minds: Remapping the World of Autism*, Roy Grinker, suggests that these changes made in the diagnostic criteria could account for 50–75 percent of the increase in prevalence rates.

A second factor that contributes to the changes in prevalence rates is the vast increase in autism awareness. This increase in awareness allows for greater identification of children who might have previously been overlooked and not diagnosed. Increased awareness also decreases the stigma of having a child with a disability, which allows families to openly seek services and become involved in treatment and educational systems. Increased awareness also means an increased awareness for professionals. As professionals become more expert at identifying autism, children can be diagnosed earlier and entered into treatment and educational programs earlier. The more children enrolled in services means the more children that are being serviced and helped. But it also means that more children can be counted when a prevalence study is being conducted.

As awareness of autism has increased, so have the treatment opportunities. Many of these treatment opportunities are expensive, but they can at times be financially covered by the school system and in some cases, by insurance coverage. However, in order to receive the financial compensation for treatment, the diagnosis of autism is necessary. This can be a crucial factor for some families and professionals, as Grinker reports in his book. He cites an example of one professional stating, facetiously, but with some truth behind it, that she would call a child a zebra if that is what it took to secure services for him.

Finally, changes in the methods used to determine and assess the number of children with a diagnosis of autism could also contribute to the rise in the prevalence rates for children with autism. Many recent studies, including the California Department of Developmental Disabilities report, utilize information based on children entering a given program, be that the special education system or regional center. In order to identify a child with a specific disorder, that disorder must first be included in the program's categorical list of diagnoses. Prior to 1991, autism wasn't listed as a specific diagnostic category in the U.S. special education system. Obviously, the disorder could not be counted if it was not listed as a possible entity. The manner in which studies of prevalence rates are conducted, therefore can have a huge impact on the observed rates of a disorder. Only if similar methods are utilized can truly accurate comparisons be made.

There are several factors that refute the notion that there is an autism epidemic, including changes in diagnostic criteria, greater awareness, and changes in epidemiological reporting and methodology. However, these factors most likely do not account for the total increase in prevalence rates that have been reported. There may be some measure of secular increase, although not at epidemic levels, in the prevalence rates of autism.

In sum, there seems to be some measure of secular increase in the rate of autism. Further, despite clear evidence of a causal genetic role, there is no specific, definitive causal pathway and mechanism identified for all cases of autism. Genes do not act in a vacuum and heritability estimates suggest there is an as yet unidentified environmental factor(s) in autism. These are props on the stage of autism and these props clearly set the scene for continued controversy about the cause of autism.

The Vaccine Controversy

The second biggest controversy concerning the etiology, or cause, of autism revolves around the role of immunizations in the cause of autism. With reports of rising prevalence rates and an "autism epidemic," many have turned their attention to toxins in the environment to identify the cause of autism. One organization maintains that there is an autism epidemic and propose that vaccines are to blame. On the organization's Web site, Generation Rescue states: "Our children are experiencing epidemics of ADD/ ADHD, Asperger's Disorder, PDD-NOS, and Autism. We believe these neurological disorders ("NDs") are environmental illnesses caused by an overload of heavy metals, live viruses, and bacteria" (Generation Rescue 2009). In order to understand this controversy, which continues today, it is essential to consider the cultural context and prevailing atmosphere of our understanding of autism.

The Contextual Factors
No Definitive Causal Genetic Mechanism, Gene-Environment Interactions, and the Lack of Identified Possible Environmental Factors

The Folstein and Rutter study in 1977 indicated that genetics are a significant factor in the etiology of autism. A follow-up twin study published in the mid-1990s by Tony Bailey and colleagues including a much larger number of twin pairs further supported the finding that genetics play a significant role in autism (Bailey et al. 1995). Based on these twin studies, heritability estimates, which are statistical estimates of the contribution of genetic and environmental factors to a disorder, were established at 91–93 percent (Freitag 2007). This suggests that approximately 90 percent of the variance of autism in the population is due to genetic factors. This is very high for a psychiatric disorder. However, that means, of course, that autism is not solely caused by genetics. There is an "environmental" factor as well.

Environmental factors in the context of heritability estimates simply mean: not genetic. Environment from a geneticist's perspective does not refer specifically to features of the natural world, such as air quality, temperature, or number of extinct species, although it could. Environment in the context of the heritability of disorders refers to factors other than genetics, which could include family environment, such as number of siblings or amount of violence in the home, or toxins in the air, or even the intra-uterine environment—the environment that the developing fetus experiences in the womb.

The identities of these environmental factors in autism have been unknown since the first twin study and remain unknown today. However, countless factors have been proposed over the years ranging from microwave signals to intra-uterine temperature changes to rainfall, to name a few. Given the multitude of possible environmental factors, many geneticists have proposed that it is essential to identify the genetic mechanisms involved in autism before attempting to identify these other risk factors.

The reason for this proposed strategy is that the phenotype for autism, that is, the observed behaviors of autism, are the result of a complex interaction between genes and environment that plays out in the brain. Imagine a grassy playing field in which 11 players with red uniforms are interacting with 11 players with green uniforms around the placement of a small, leather ball into two opposing nets. The result of this complex interaction is the game of soccer. If we removed the colored jerseys it might take the uninformed viewer some time to determine the rules of the game. But, by putting colored jerseys on just one team, it makes a significant difference in helping the novice sports watcher figure out what is happening in the game. Now imagine that there are thousands of players on the field, hundreds of balls, and tens of nets. And there are no colored jerseys. This is akin to the complexity of autism. Given the complexity of the interaction in autism, by shedding light on one side of the complex interaction, the genetic contribution, scientists believe it will be easier to then identify how the environmental contribution interacts to result in autism. This has been the strategy of the late 1990s and early 2000s in exploring causal factors in autism.

Genetic studies have employed a number of technological and statistical strategies relying on advances in genetics to identify the risk genes for autism. In the 1990s, genome wide linkage scans became possible due to advances in genetic technologies. In genome wide linkage scans blood is collected from each family member in a "multiplex family"—a family in which more than one person has autism. Most often the participating families are families for which two children have autism. Then, through complicated genetic processes and statistical analyses, scientists identify regions in the genetic code that have potential to contain genes related to autism. These initial studies published in the late 1990s and early 2000s clearly indicated that the genetics of autism were not as straightforward and simple as the recessive and dominant transmission methods that Gregor Mendel discussed with his peas in the 1800s. While many potential "hotspots" throughout the genome have been identified, a number of possible candidate genes have been suggested, and a number of theoretical genetic transmission processes have been proposed, no definitive genetic causal mechanism has been identified yet for the majority of cases of autism.

Without a definitive genetic mechanism, it is impossible to rule out which of the possible billions of environmental factors might be playing a role in autism. This leaves almost any of these environmental factors open to debate. The lack of a definitive genetic mechanism for autism, coupled with the fact that genes do not operate without input from the environment, has set the stage for controversies about the environmental contribution to autism. However, there are other factors to consider in the context of the current controversy.

Timing of Symptom Onset

Another important contributing factor related to the current vaccine controversy concerns the timing with which symptoms emerge in autism. The mean age in the United States at which a child is diagnosed with an ASD is estimated at 5.1 years of age (Wiggins, Baio, and Rice 2006) while the median age 5.7 years old (Shattuck et al. 2009). However, the age at which a disorder such as autism is diagnosed indicates little about the biology or even about the emergence of symptoms. The age of diagnosis reflects a combination of factors including how old the child is when parents first note problems, when the consulted professional, most often a pediatrician, considers the problems worthy of referral, and when a child is finally able to be evaluated by a specialist who can make a formal diagnosis. This process can take more than two years in some cases. In fact, research indicates that parents most often report problems with their child's development in the first two years of life indicating a long time indeed, between recognizing difficulties and receiving a diagnosis.

The symptoms that parents most often first report noting are delays and difficulties with language and communication as well as abnormalities in social responsiveness. However, in an estimated one quarter of children with autism, development appears to develop typically for the first year of life, followed by a regression in language, social and other skills (Wiggins, Rice, and Baio 2009). On average, parents report that the regression occurs around 18 months of age. When parents talk about these early years, comments from parents attending the University of Washington Autism Center clinic include, "he just wasn't talking as much as his older sister and I thought, well, maybe his sister is just doing his talking for him . . . she loves to talk, you know." Or, another parent has said, "Paul just didn't seem very interested in me or anyone else when he was a baby. After he learned to walk around a year of age, he just wandered around the living room in circles not very interested in us." Or, yet another parent has said, "In the first year of his life, Joey, seemed just like a typical baby. He cooed, babbled, had even started saying mama, dada, and ball. But then just before a year and a half, he stopped being so interested in others and stopped making sounds altogether. We didn't know what was happening" (R. Bernier, unpublished data).In typical development, many children begin using single words, such as mama and dada around the first birthday and short phrases shortly thereafter. However, there is a large range in the age at which children begin to speak. Practice parameters suggest that parents consult a physician if a child is not using single words by 16 months of age and two word phrases by 24 months (Filipek et al. 1999). Also typical development social skills, such as orienting to your name or using a point to show something of interest, only emerge in the second half of the first year of life. What this means is that if development is progressing abnormally, it is difficult to notice until after a child is old enough to demonstrate the skills in the first place.

Parents first start noticing abnormalities in their child's development in the first two years of life, at some point after the typical age that skills should first emerge. When parents first start noticing delays, or a regression in skills, often the first thing that parents do is review recent adverse events in the child's life to identify a potential cause of the difficulty. During the first two years of life, children receive a number of vaccinations and crying, fatigue, and occasionally fevers, are the child's response to the pokes. Vaccines are easy targets for blame because they are an easily identifiable adverse event in a baby's life that happens around the time that abnormalities (or regressions) are first observed in autism.

But there are other factors to consider besides the rise in autism prevalence rates, the lack of a definitive genetic mechanism, the lack of identified environmental factors, and the correlated timing between symptom presentation and vaccine schedule in the current controversy. Several specific events have fueled the vaccine controversy.

Events in the Controversy
The Initial Study
The first study to suggest a link between vaccines and autism was one published in 1998 in England's most prestigious medical journal, the *Lancet*. (Wakefield et al. 1998). The team of authors, led by Andrew Wakefield, a physician at the Royal Free Hospital in London, concluded that there was a connection between gastrointestinal disorders and autism. In a sample of eight children with autism and four children with autism symptoms with gastrointestinal disease, they reported a regression in skills following the measles-mumps-rubella (MMR) immunization. In the final paragraph of the manuscript, the authors state: "We have identified a chronic enterocolitis in children that may be related to neuropsychiatric dysfunction. In most cases, onset of symptoms was after

measles, mumps, and rubella immunisation" (Wakefield et al. 1998, p. 641). During the press conference held on the day of publication of the manuscript, Dr. Wakefield proposed that the MMR vaccine may be causing the gastrointestinal inflammation in these children with autism. With the press conference and publication, the curtain was raised on the controversy regarding the vaccines and autism.

The press conference garnered immediate media attention and parents and families responded. In the 10 years since the publication in the *Lancet*, the *New York Times* alone has published almost 4,000 letters, articles, or editorials regarding autism and vaccines. Following the publication of the manuscript, the immunization rates for the MMR vaccine dropped precipitously in England. One year after the press conference, the online version of the newspaper the *Guardian* in England reported on a study highlighting concerns of the possible return of a rubella epidemic. "Britain could face a new rubella epidemic with devastating effects on unborn babies if parents continue to shun the MMR vaccine, according to a report by child health specialists published yesterday" (Boseley 1999). In 2008, the *New York Times* reported "Measles Cases Grow in Number, and Officials Blame Parents' Fear of Autism" (Harris 2008). And, as reported in the *Times* in February of 2009 (Lister 2009), the Health Protection Agency in the United Kingdom indicated that in 2008 there was a 36 percent increase in the numbers of children infected with measles with 1,348 new cases reported. This is in stark contrast to 56 cases of measles reported in 1998. There was clearly a significant response to the claims that the MMR vaccine was linked to autism spurred by the first and only paper to publish a relationship between the MMR vaccine and autism.

The study that generated so much attention and had a substantial impact on parental behavior also generated a second flurry of controversy six years later. In 2004, the *Lancet* published statements from 10 of Dr. Wakefield's 12 coauthors on the paper retracting the conclusions from the 1998 publication (Horton 2004; Murch et al. 2004). As reported in the March 7, 2004, issue of the *Sunday Times,* the *Lancet* retraction followed an investigation by a reporter from the *Sunday Times* who found that Dr. Wakefield had been given approximately $100,000 by a personal injury lawyer (Rogers 2004). The lawyer was involved in a class-action lawsuit against a pharmaceutical company that manufactured vaccinations, such as the MMR vaccine. Further, the journalist reported that several of the research participants were clients of the personal injury lawyer and these families had a financial interest in identifying a link between the MMR vaccine and autism. Subsequent investigation, as reported in Paul Offit's *Autism's False Prophets*, suggested that this figure of $100,000 was a significant underestimate of the amount of money given to Dr. Wakefield for research to link the MMR vaccine and autism (Offit 2008). This represented a significant conflict of interest for Dr. Wakefield, and the *Lancet* editors noted that he failed to report this conflict of interest when submitting the manuscript for publication.

Conflicts of interest are expected to happen in science and research and are one of the reasons that submitted manuscripts are subjected to close peer review during the scientific process. Before a researcher can publish a manuscript with scientific findings, the manuscript must undergo careful scrutiny by experts in the field who then recommend to the chief editor of a scientific journal to publish, reject, or accept with revisions the submitted manuscript. During this process the methodology of the study is reviewed for accuracy, the results are assessed for veracity, and conclusions are examined to ensure they follow directly from the results and methodology. Additionally, conflicts of interest are considered to rule out the possibility of bias in the research. However, in the case of the 1998 manuscript, Dr. Wakefield failed to report this conflict of interest to the journal and to all of his coauthors.

Failing to cite a conflict of interest does not inherently mean that the underlying science is faulty or that the conclusions are inaccurate. But, it does mean that the scientists conducting the research may inadvertently overlook findings or reach flawed conclusions as a result. The reviewers for the 1998 *Lancet* paper reviewed the study and determined that based upon what the authors wrote, the methodology was sound, the results viable, and the conclusions reasonable for publication. However, in 2004, the *Lancet* editorial board considered this omission of the conflict of interest to be significant in the case of the Wakefield study and retracted the paper (Horton 2004).

Supporters of the MMR vaccine and autism connection have also argued that a conflict of interest within the medical community has promoted the continued use of vaccines. Bloggers have posted a range of proposed conflicts including suggestions that the *Sunday Times* was receiving special funds by the medical establishment to discredit the link between vaccines and autism and that the numerous research studies finding no link between vaccines and autism were, in fact, funded by pharmaceutical companies, thereby suggestive of a conflict of interest. Clearly conflicts of interest can generate a bias in conclusions that can be drawn in a scientific inquiry. This is why the peer review process is essential, but it is also why a second component of the scientific method, independent replication, is invaluable.

An important second step in the scientific process, following the peer review of a research study, is independent replication of those findings. That is, in science, scientific conclusions from a research study, such as the MMR vaccine causes autism, must be replicated by other scientists who work independently from the original scientists to lend credibility to that finding. Through this process of using similar methodology to replicate findings or by addressing the question using complementary methodologies, advances in science are slowly and carefully made. This process is essential so that only true findings are accepted and become part of scientific knowledge. In the more than a decade since the 1998 publication linking MMR and autism, the finding has yet to be replicated despite numerous attempts to reproduce the findings. Indeed, many studies using similar methods and complementary epidemiological methods have reported no link between the MMR vaccine and autism (Schreibman 2005).

There was a final controversy surrounding the 1998 *Lancet* publication in the spring of 2009. Further investigation by Brian Deer of the *Sunday Times* in London of medical records and eyewitness testimony suggested that the data presented in the 1998 publication was fixed to produce the desired result (Deer 2009). Medical records were presented to the Medical Research Council in the United Kingdom and the investigation revealed that many of the symptoms the children reportedly experienced in the publication differed from what was noted in their medical records. Further, the symptoms reportedly noted following vaccination, were found to actually be present prior to the vaccination. This suggests that the vaccines in these cases could not be causal as the symptoms were observed *before* ever having the vaccine.

Dr. Wakefield provided a rebuttal to this recent investigation in the form of annotations to the letter he received by journalist Deer two days prior to the printing of the story in February 2009. Dr. Wakefield titled his response, "In his desperation, Deer gets it wrong once again," and in his annotations he states that he did not alter the data and that the purpose of the paper was not to intentionally link the vaccine to autism, but to present a syndrome of gastrointestinal illness and developmental disability. Dr. Wakefield ends his annotated rebuttal with: "I did not 'create' a scare but rather, I responded to a scare that parents brought to my attention. To have ignored their concerns would have been professional negligence" (Wakefield 2009, p. 4).

Evidence of Harm and Autism's False Prophets

Two books stand out in the controversy between vaccines and autism. In 2005, David Kirby, a journalist, shared the stories of parents of children with autism combined with commentary and excerpts from the scientific community and government officials in a book titled, *Evidence of Harm: Mercury in Vaccines and the Autism Epidemic: A Medical Controversy* (Kirby 2005). The *New York Times* book review "What Caused the Autism Epidemic?" commends David Kirby's ability to present the complicated information and jargon related to the controversy and to describe the theoretical process by which vaccines could cause autism, but highlights that readers "might welcome a summary" of the mainstream research findings, which are not presented in the book (Morrice 2005, p. 20).

Evidence of Harm is based on several years of research by Kirby and presents family stories of all too common challenges to receiving an appropriate diagnosis of autism. Kirby presents the controversy including Dr. Wakefield's proposal of an MMR vaccine and autism connection and he reviews the parent group-led proposal that it is a compound called thimerosal, the mercury containing preservative used to bind the vaccines, that is the causal agent in the etiology of autism. A galvanization for many parents was the American Academy of Pediatrics' statement to request the removal of thimerosal from vaccines in 1999 (American Academy of Pediatrics 1999). This event is presented in his book and served as the basis for its title. The issued report, for many parents, served as evidence that thimerosal was the culprit in the controversy. In the Academy report, researchers indicated that babies were receiving doses of ethylmercury in thimerosal in vaccines that exceeded the federal limitations of a different, yet chemically related compound, methylmercury. The authors of the report, however, concluded that there was "no evidence of harm" of using the thimerosal preservative in the vaccines.

In the years subsequent to the removal of thimerosal from vaccines, a variety of peer reviewed, scientific studies were conducted. In 2004, the Institute of Medicine in the United States issued a statement concluding there was no link between thimerosal and incidence of autism (Institute of Medicine 2004). Kirby indicated in his book that the definitive answer would be found soon after the publication of the book. In 2007, data from California's Department of Developmental Disabilities rang in the verdict. By 2001, the preservative had been removed from all infant vaccines (and remains only in some multiple dose flu vaccines), and, by the time of the report, six years had passed since the removal of the preservative. Given that children are generally diagnosed with autism by six years of age, children not exposed to the preservative could be compared to children who had been exposed to the preservative. It was a simple matter of comparing the population of children born prior to 2001, when thimerosal was included in the vaccine, to those children born after the removal of the preservative. If thimerosal were truly the causal agent, then a drastic reduction in the cases of autism should be seen. The California data, calculated and tallied in a report released in January 2008, showed that rates of autism had not decreased but, in fact, continued to increase (Schechter and Grether 2008).

Sally Bernard, a parent of a child with autism and autism advocate, commented on the findings. She stated that the report indicated that there were significant environmental factors in the etiology of autism and did not rule out thimerosal as one of them (DeNoon 2008). Sally Bernard cofounded Coalition of SafeMinds (Sensible Action for Ending Mercury-Induced Neurological Disorders) with Lyn Redwood, also a parent and advocate whose story was told in Kirby's book. They were the first to propose the thimerosal-autism connection in a publication in the journal *Medical Hypothesis* (Bernard et al. 2001).

These same events are also told in another book published concerning this controversy. Paul Offit's *Autism's False Prophets: Bad Science, Risky Medicine, and the Search for a Cure* went to press in 2008. Similar to David Kirby's *Evidence of Harm*, Dr. Offit presents the vaccine autism controversy incorporating media commentary, firsthand accounts, parental insight, and data. Counter to *Evidence of Harm*, Dr. Offit's book underscores that there is no connection between vaccines and autism and he couches his conclusion in a description of the context that gave rise to the controversy, as has been reviewed above. As the chief of Infectious Diseases and director of the Vaccine Education Center at the Children's Hospital of Philadelphia and the Maurice R. Hilleman Professor of Vaccinology and professor of pediatrics at the University of Pennsylvania School of Medicine, Dr. Offit presented his book from a position of great authority in the medical community. Dr. Offit has been the recipient of numerous awards, including Jonas Salk Award from the Association for Professionals in Infection Control and Epidemiology for coinventing the rotavirus vaccine RotaTeq. It is precisely because of these awards and his established history in the medical community that his book has received criticism.

Proponents of the vaccine autism link attribute Dr. Offit's stance that vaccines do not play a causal role in autism to a conflict of interest of financial incentives from pharmaceutical companies. Proponents claim that because Dr. Offit conducts funded research into vaccines he has a conflict of interest that makes his conclusions invalid and that leads him to say vaccines are safe. Dr. Offit's rebuttal is simply "the reason I say vaccines don't cause autism is that they don't" (Offit 2008, p. xvii).

Subsequent to the publication of these two books that received a great deal of attention from both "sides" of the controversy, a final event in the drama unfolded in the court system.

The Vaccine Injury Compensation Program

The vaccine injury compensation program is a federally funded program to provide financial compensation to families following an adverse reaction to vaccination. Through this program started in 1986, families can quickly receive financial compensation of $900,000 in a very short time provided it can be definitively demonstrated that the injury was caused by the vaccination. This program was started to alleviate the number of lawsuits directed against vaccine makers that in the mid-1980s threatened to end vaccine manufacturing. While this program does not entirely protect vaccine makers, because if families are dissatisfied with rulings pharmaceutical companies can be sued in state courts, it has dramatically reduced the number of lawsuits.

Between 1999 and 2007, more than 5,000 families made claims that vaccines caused their child's autism. This number overpowered the vaccine injury compensation court and as a result the court decided to address the claims like a class-action lawsuit. Called the Omnibus Autism Proceeding, the trial began in the summer of 2007 and focused on three specific cases.

On February 12, 2009, the courts revealed their verdict. After reviewing the testimony concerning the three cases and including expert witnesses from both sides, the three judges that comprise the panel determined that for each case there was no evidence that the children's autism was caused the MMR vaccine and thimerosal (*Cedillo v. Secretary of Health and Human Services Case No. 98-916v* 2009; *Hazelhurst v. Secretary of Health and Human Services Case No. 03-654v* 2009; *Snyder v. Secretary of Health and Human Services Case No. 01-162v* 2009).

All three verdicts in this omnibus proceeding in the history of the vaccine act dealt a sharp blow to the theory claiming that vaccines cause autism. Yet, there is one additional case that warrants discussion in this controversy: Hannah Poling. In the fall of 2007, the Vaccine Injury Compensation Program compensated the family concluding that her injuries were linked to the vaccine. CNN reported on March 7, 2008, the "underlying illness that had predisposed her to symptoms of autism was "significantly aggravated" by the vaccinations she received" (CNN 2008). Hannah Poling's parents describe a regression and loss of skills in Hannah and onset of autism symptoms. In addition to autism, Hannah was also diagnosed with a mitochondrial disorder. Mitochondria are the energy manufacturers of the cell and dysfunction of the mitochondria can occur in a variety of cell types: skin, brain, heart and lung. As a result, the symptoms of mitochondrial disorder vary greatly and can at times go undetected. There are only a few known cases of mitochondrial disorder and autism. Chief science officer at Autism Speaks Dr. Geraldine Dawson commented on the ruling: "Vaccines stimulate the immune system, which may put stress on the cell function of a child who has asymptomatic mitochondrial dysfunction or disorder such that the child now shows increased symptoms. In an extreme case, the symptoms could involve regression and symptoms of autism" (Dawson 2008). As reported in *Time* magazine online, the director of the Centers for Disease Control and Prevention, Dr. Julie Gerberding, underscored, "the government has made absolutely no statement about indicating that vaccines are the cause of autism, as this would be a complete mischaracterization of any of the science that we have at our disposal today" (Wallis 2008). The federal vaccine court found that the underlying cellular disorder, the mitochondrial disorder, was aggravated by vaccines and that in this particular case, symptoms of autism resulted. Contrary to the omnibus proceedings, this specific finding has encouraged those advocates of an autism vaccine connection.

The scene was set and specific events took place to fuel the vaccine-autism controversy. Despite scientific evidence indicating that no causal link between vaccines and autism, the controversy persists. In part this is due to the context surrounding the controversy: the lack of a definitive causal mechanism for autism leaves the door open for speculations about putative causes, including the role of vaccinations. Further, the onset of symptoms and timing of vaccines make vaccines a clear choice to consider. There is also a rising prevalence rate of autism that science suggests is not at epidemic levels, but does indicate that there may be some increase in the rate of cases. Finally, the persistence of this controversy is in part due to the vast array of information that is available to families. The amount of information on the Internet regarding autism is staggering. An Internet Google search of the word "autism" returned 18,300,000 hits at the time that this book was written. In comparison, the word "schizophrenia," a psychiatric disorder identified and diagnosed many years before autism, returned only 10,200,000 hits. Unfortunately, not all that information has undergone scientific scrutiny. But, it is printed; and when information is printed, some credibility seems to be automatically lent to it. This means that families are presented with not only a vast array of information, but also a vast array of misinformation and it can be very challenging to discern the two.

In April 2009 on the *Huffington Post*, the actor Jim Carrey wrote about his belief that vaccines could cause autism and suggested that decisions regarding vaccines were based on money not safety. He wrote: "With vaccines being the fastest growing division of the pharmaceutical industry, isn't it possible that profits may play a part in the decision-making? That the vaccine program is becoming more of a profit engine than a means of prevention?" (Carrey 2009). One year prior, in April 2008, the actress Jenny McCarthy stated, "We believe autism is an environmental illness. Vaccines are not the only environmental trigger, but we do think they play a major role" (McCarthy and Carrey 2008). Both these statements are readily available to Google searchers across the world. It is important that they are available, but what is equally important is that readers know how to assess the accuracy of what is written. Science relies on the scientific method to disprove hypotheses (the scientific method cannot prove—only disprove), and it requires replication to ensure the accuracy of findings. Further, before any scientific results are published, other scientists painstakingly review the researcher's manuscript to ensure the accuracy and veracity of what has been written. Through this process, accurate information can be translated to the public. It is important (and often uncommon) that information gleaned through this process be as available to the public as the information that is presented via movie stars' statements. At this point, science has been unable to compete.

Despite the controversy regarding the role of vaccines in autism, there is forward momentum in the field. The field of autism genetics has grown exponentially in the past two to three years and innovative new technologies and elucidating discoveries are made on a regular basis at this point in time. New research into the interaction between genetics and environment is also on the rise. However, definitive answers from the genetics community and reports from collaborative work between scientists from multiple disciplines clarifying gene environment pathways in autism are essential to buy-in from the general public. Such advances and answers will hopefully even the playing field and allow science to better compete with alluring statements from celebrities. The end goal to all of this exploration into true causes of autism is to recommend and implement the most effective treatments, interventions, and, perhaps some day, preventions of autism. However, autism treatment research to date has also been plagued by controversy.

Controversies Surrounding the Treatment of Autism

As heated as the debate has been concerning the cause of autism, discussion and controversy has also afflicted autism treatment. Similarly to the debate concerning the etiology of autism, there are a number of factors that make the concerns around autism intervention ripe for controversy.

One of the reasons that controversy surrounds treatments for autism is that there is no specific known cause for autism. There are most likely many causes that lead to the pattern of behaviors we term autism (Geschwind 2009). When the cause of a disorder is known, then the appropriate intervention can be assigned. If a person arrives at the doctor's office with congestion and headache, there are a number of things that could possibly have caused the pattern of symptoms. By identifying the cause, a doctor can prescribe the appropriate treatment. For example, if the congestion and pain was caused by a viral infection, then the prescription may be rest and lots of fluids. If the symptoms are the manifestations of a bacterial sinus infection, then perhaps, a course of antibiotics would be the appropriate treatment. Or yet, if the congestion and headache are caused by seasonal allergies, then perhaps the best course of action would be an antihistamine.

However, even with the etiology of autism identified this still may not necessarily advance treatment. In approximately 10–20 percent of cases of autism, the specific cause is known, but this has not advanced treatment options significantly (Geschwind 2009). Even though advanced and new treatment options may not necessarily result from an identified etiology of autism, by identifying the causal pathway, treatments can be validated or refuted by virtue of their proposed mechanism.

A second reason that controversies persist regarding autism treatments is that currently the only treatment that has been empirically demonstrated to be effective in treating children with autism is behavioral intervention based upon methods of Applied Behavioral Analysis (ABA) (Schreibman 2005). There are no medication treatments for autism although there are medication treatments for associated behaviors such as the management of aggressive or self-injurious behavior (Research Units on Pediatric Psychopharmacology Autism Network 2002). Behavioral intervention for autism is time intensive—some programs include 40 hours of repetitive practice each week for the child. Children progress with ABA treatment programs, but progress is slow and can take months or even years to see noticeable gains. This can be painstaking for a parent wanting and waiting for his or her child to successfully interact with the world around. Additionally, the cost of intervention can be staggering, with current estimates suggesting approximately $25,000 per year of ABA treatment. Currently, for most families this treatment is paid out of pocket as most insurance companies do not provide coverage. However, efforts are underway by lobbying groups to address this problem and some states have made substantial gains in intervention coverage. The considerable time requirement, the slow pace of progress, and the overwhelming financial burden limit the feasibility of behavioral intervention for many families.

Finally, similar to availability of information regarding the causes of autism, so too is there a vast array of information (and misinformation) about treatment possibilities for autism. In this complex arena of statistics, figures, anecdotal reports, case studies, and experimental studies, there are thousands of treatment options, ranging from empirically supported behavioral treatments to treatments that have actually caused significant harm to children. Even among the behaviorally based treatments—termed *efficacious* treatments, there are a multitude of names and abbreviations, such as PRT (pivotal response training), ABA, and ESDM (early start Denver model), so that it is difficult to navigate through the options.

Parents receiving a first-time diagnosis of autism for their child experience the diagnostic process in as many ways as there are people, but for many, receiving the diagnosis is an emotionally turbulent time. Faced with that emotional struggle, the multitude of options available makes it difficult for parents to mire through the mountain of information regarding treatment options. Many clinicians encourage families to consider treatment options through an analytic 2 × 2 matrix (Cohen and Eisenberg 2002). On the left side of the matrix, one considers the safety: yes the treatment is safe, or no it is not. On the top of the matrix, one considers the effectiveness: yes the treatment is effective, or no it is not. By comparing the four cells of the matrix, the appropriate course of action regarding that intervention can be determined. If the treatment is safe and effective, it is recommended. If it safe but not effective, it can be tolerated. If it is effective but unsafe, it can be monitored closely or discouraged. Clearly, if a treatment is ineffective and unsafe, it should be discouraged. The application of the treatment decision matrix to the four treatments implicated in controversies that are described below may be a useful exercise.

As yet, there are no identified causes of autism that can direct or guide promising interventions and the only empirically supported treatment is often perceived to be slow, time consuming, and costly. There is also significant difficulty in navigating information and misinformation available to families regarding intervention options. Combined with a parent's driving desire to do what is going to help his or her child, it is no surprise that controversies exist concerning autism treatment. There have been four specific controversies in autism treatment in the recent years. The controversies include the touting of facilitated communication as a miracle cure, the media attention over secretin, the use of biomedical interventions, such as chelation, and the use of dietary interventions in autism.

Facilitated Communication

Facilitated communication (FC) was an augmentative communication technique developed in Australia in the 1970s. It was originally developed to assist individuals with cerebral palsy to express themselves based on the belief that with additional support, individuals would be able to demonstrate their true capacities. In facilitated communication an individual is seated at a keyboard or other letter-displaying instrument. A facilitator provides support for the communicator by holding his or her hand, arm, or elbow as the communicator selects or points to letters on the keyboard or visual display. Through this facilitation, the individual is then able to communicate in a manner that is purported to be more effective and reflective of his or her true abilities.

In 1990 Douglas Biklen, a professor of special education at Syracuse University in New York, returned from Melbourne Australia where he had seen Rosemary Crossley, the teacher who developed the program based on her work with cerebral palsy, model the technique. He introduced the technique in the United States, and it quickly became widespread so much so that in 1993 he developed the Facilitated Communication Institute at Syracuse. Through facilitation it was reported that nonverbal children with autism were suddenly conveying sophisticated messages showing a strong grasp of grammatical structure and abstract conceptual understanding. The treatment was far less expensive than behavioral intervention and produced results much more quickly while offering families hope and promise of success for their children. Through the facilitators, children who had never produced single words in their lifetime remarkably relayed long sought after messages of social connection, such as "I love you, Mommy," and provided parents with a window into the apparently impenetrable minds of their children.

Unfortunately, FC took hold before any analysis of its effectiveness could be made; there were harmful consequences as a result. In *The Science and Fiction of Autism,* Laura Schreibman recounts receiving countless calls regarding the efficacy of the intervention but being unable to report anything other than a healthy skepticism because she had not seen any research on it yet (Schreibman 2005). Prompted by allegations of sexual abuse made through FC by children with autism, prosecutors needed to do a thorough examination of Facilitated Communication.

Paul Offit describes the experience of the Wheaton family as the impetus that set in motion the critical examination of FC (Offit 2008). Betsy Wheaton, a 17-year-old girl with autism, reported through the use of FC that she was being sexually abused by her parents, grandparents, and brother. Similar allegations were being reported throughout the country using FC. This prompted prosecutors and scientists alike to determine the way in which FC produced its results. A simple experiment was developed and conducted by scientists with no conflict of interest in the results. In the basic experiment, the table was divided in two with a screen such that the facilitator could only see her side of the table and the child communicator only his or her side. Then the facilitator and child were shown various pictures that the other could not see. Sometimes the child and facilitator were shown the same picture, while other times the pictures differed. As Offit describes, when Betsy and her facilitator were shown a picture of a key, Betsy typed in the word *key* with her facilitator. When Betsy was shown a picture of a cup and her facilitator shown a picture of a hat, Betsy typed the word *hat*. The results were clear: Betsy's facilitator was doing the communicating.

This same pattern was observed over and over again using this experimental paradigm and a similar paradigm. In the alternative test paradigm, the child was removed from the presence of the facilitator, shown some information that the facilitator had no access to, and then asked to indicate what was seen or heard upon return to the facilitator and the FC device. Regardless of which experimental paradigm was used, the results were the same. The facilitators were doing the communicating, not the child. Follow up analyses suggested that the facilitators were not doing this maliciously or with evil intent. Indeed, psychologist Donald Wegner reported on a series of five studies examining the phenomena of ideomotor effects and concluded that facilitators of FC were not intending to mislead or direct the communicator's behavior but did so unconsciously (Wegner Fuller, and Sparrow 2003).

The research in the mid-1990s dealt a significant blow to the FC movement and a number of national organizations, including the American Speech and Hearing Association, the Association for Behavioral Analysis, the American Association on Mental Retardation and the American Academy of Child and Adolescent Psychiatry, have provided position statements indicating their failure to support FC due to its lack of scientific validity. Despite this, the Facilitated Communication Institute exists today, and proponents of the technique continue to promote its use. The parent-based nonprofit organization Autism National Committee (or AutCom) issued a policy statement in 2008 regarding FC. It states, "It is the policy of the Autism National Committee that everyone has something to say and a right to say it. Facilitated Communication is one accepted and valid way in which individuals with autism can exercise their right to say what they have to say" (Autism National Committee 2008, p. 1).

In summary, the scientific research suggests that FC is not an effective treatment as it is the facilitators that are communicating *for* the individual with the disability, not the individual with autism. This is reflected in the position statements of several national organizations. Additionally, it has become increasingly clear that FC could be considered harmful. Firstly, the widespread reports of abuse resulted in significant devastation to many families despite the subsequent drop in charges. In most cases the allegations were unjustified and yet led to the removal of children from their home and incarceration of family members. The resulting impact on the family's financial and community standing as well as emotional and mental health was considerable. Secondly, time spent engaging in FC is time not spent engaging in treatments that are effective and shown to be helpful for children with autism. Given the importance of intervening as early as possible, time spent on treatments shown to be ineffective can be considered harmful. Thirdly, the diversion of funds to FC programs from efficacious treatment programs restricts intervention options. Finally, the destroyed hopes, promises, and dreams of families who thought FC was helping their children could be considered significant harm (Schreibman 2005).

Secretin

While the controversy over FC took center stage in the mid-1990s, it shared the stage in the late 1990s with a second controversial treatment that also proved to be ineffective. In October 1998, *Dateline* aired a segment reporting on a miraculous recovery by a young child with autism, named Parker Beck (Pauley 1998). The program described five-year-old Parker's early development and loss of skills just after he turned two. Following what his parents described as happy and healthy early development, he lost his social interest, smiles, speech, and became more irritable and began spinning repetitively. In addition, his parents reported that he had persistent diarrhea and stomach pain. The program described the Beck's family struggles with finding treatment for Parker's diagnosis of autism and their chance encounter with a pediatric gastroenterologist. While assessing Parker, Dr. Horvath conducted an endoscopy and administered secretin to test Parker's pancreatic functioning. Secretin is a peptide hormone produced by cells in the small intestine. Soon after the visit, Victoria, Parker's mother, reported dramatic improvement in Parker's symptoms. His gastrointestinal difficulties subsided and he began making more eye contact and using more language.

The Beck family tried to identify what during the procedure could have effected the change and after pouring over the records; they concluded that the secretin that was used as a diagnostic tool could have been the catalyst for Parker's change. However, they struggled to find a source for secretin as the Federal Drug Administration (FDA) had not approved the use of secretin for anything other than what Dr. Horvath had used it for, a diagnostic aid. Doctors were unwilling to prescribe secretin "off-label," for a use not approved by the FDA. During the time the Becks were searching for another source of secretin, Parker stopped improving. Over a year later, they found a doctor willing to administer secretin and they reported seeing signs of Parker's improvement again.

After the Beck family's experience with secretin and Parker, they contacted the Autism Research Institute, founded by Dr. Rimland. He shared the family's experience with other families. A family in California was intrigued and mirrored the procedure with a local gastroenterologist. The second family also observed the same result. A third family had a similar experience and so Dr. Horvath and colleagues published their findings in 1998 (Horvath et al. 1998). The *Dateline* program shared this story highlighting that is was a treatment pioneered by parents, not the medical or research.

Following the airing of the program, autism clinics and research programs received countless calls from families requesting information about secretin. There was an outpouring of parental interest in utilizing secretin as a treatment for autism although practitioners had no experience in using the hormone in this manner. The medical community was not prepared to meet the patient-driven demand for this treatment that had no empirical support. On a pediatrician Listserve, one physician posted two days after the *Dateline* airing: "Anyone care to comment re: the dateline show related to using secretin for autism? Anyone with any experience with the medication? Any adverse side effects? Any published research or pending research?" The next posting was a response, "Two of my patients have already asked me about it. Our local Pediatric Gastroenterology unit is besieged. They are trying to organize a well controlled study" (Shapiro 1998).

There was a rush on secretin and at the time only one manu-facturer of the peptide hormone existed. As a result, costs went through the roof and families spent thousands of dollars acquir-ing the hormone and finding doctors to prescribe it. An article was published in the *Ladies Home Journal* regarding the positive experi-ence of an eight-year-old receiving a secretin injection (McLellan 1999). This fueled parents' hopes for the treatment and wishes to have access to the hormone. It was a challenging time for families as they waited for research results.

In December of 1999, a group of researchers published the results of their controlled study of 56 children in the prestigious *New England Journal of Medicine* (Sandler et al. 1999). In this study, half of the children were randomly assigned to a course of secretin and half were randomly assigned to a placebo, an injection of salt water. The random assignment assures that any differences ob-served between groups is not due to some other factor related to the assignment of each research participant to a specific group. In the four weeks following the treatment parents, teachers, and clinicians observed the children's behavior using a variety of mea-sures. Importantly, none of the parents, teachers or clinicians rat-ing the children's behavior knew if they received the secretin or placebo. There were no differences between the groups in their be-haviors following the injection. Interestingly, both groups showed improvement in the social and communicative abilities in this study. The authors concluded that secretin was no more effective in reducing symptoms of autism than salt water, but demonstrated the power of wanting children to improve following a medical procedure.

In the several years following this initial publication, 15 con-trolled, blind studies all concluded that secretin was an ineffective treatment for autism. A controlled study is one in which random assignment and other measures are used to ensure that findings are related to the experimental manipulation and not anything else, like normal improvement over time. A blind study is one in which those observing and rating child behaviors were "blind" to what treatment the child received: secretin or placebo. Controls are essential in studies such as these so that other factors do not lead a scientist to conclude that a treatment is effective when it is not. In four of these 15 studies, a subgroup of children with gastroin-testinal symptoms reportedly demonstrated improvement in their GI symptoms, but these findings have not been replicated by a separate research group (Sturmey 2005).

In the quarterly newsletter published by the Autism Research International, Dr. Stephen Edelson reports that despite the many published findings, more research is needed for secretin and highlights that the Autism Research Institute has collected surveys from parents of 468 individuals who have had secretin injections. Forty-four percent of these respondents report seeing an improvement in their child's behavior (Edelson 2008).

The *Dateline* story, the *Ladies Home Journal* story, and the initial Horvath publication fueled excitement about secretin as a treatment for autism. The scientific community responded with well-designed studies to examine its effectiveness. Again, science moved slowly and in the process families spent thousands of dollars pursuing a treatment option that the research had demonstrated to be effective. Well-designed, controlled studies indicate that secretin is not an effective treatment for autism and suggest that limited adverse effects have been noted, but this is not definitive. The FDA has only approved secretin's use as a diagnostic tool for pancreatic functioning, not for treatment.

Chelation

A third area of controversy in the treatment of autism involves the use of chelation. Chelation was a process first developed after World War I as a method to remove poisonous gas from an exposed individual. The chelating agent was used to bind with the metal, arsenic, on which the poisonous gas was based. When the chelating agent bound to the arsenic, it formed water-soluble molecules that could pass through the bloodstream and be excreted from the system through the kidneys and liver. The original chelating agents had significant side effects (Bell 1977).

Following the initial introduction of chelation as a process to remove metal-based poisonous gas from the body, the process had been proposed as a method of removing other heavy metals, such as lead, mercury and also calcium. Following World War II, chelation was used in the treatment of lead poisoning, but as overall cases of lead poisoning have decreased over the years, so has chelation's use. That is, until it was proposed as a treatment for autism, for which it has been used as an alternative treatment without the approval and recommendation of the medical and scientific community.

Chelation was proposed as a treatment for autism in accordance with the theory that autism is the result of mercury poisoning. In the study by Bernard et al. (2001) published in *Medical Hypotheses,* the authors suggest that given their hypothesis that mercury causes autism, chelation may be an appropriate treatment. They write, "With perhaps 1 in 150 children now diagnosed with ASD, development of HgP-related treatments, such as chelation, would prove beneficial for this large and seemingly growing population" (Bernard et al. 2001, p. 467). This paper representing the hypothesis of mercury's causal role in autism and the proposal that chelation is, therefore, a viable treatment has been cited consistently by proponents of chelation for autism. A paper published in the *Journal of American Physicians and Surgeons* (Bradstreet et al. 2003) reported on differential rates of mercury excretions between 221 children with autism and 18 typical children following an oral chelation treatment. The authors concluded that the findings were suggestive of evidence of mercury poisoning, which they surmised as related to vaccine exposure and that chelation was an effective means of assessing this.

Neither of the above publications provides scientific evidence for chelation's effectiveness as a treatment for autism. In a letter published in the British Journal of Medicine, Dr. Sinha and colleagues state, "there is no compelling evidence to suggest that chelation therapy is an effective treatment for autism. A review of Medline (1966 to April 2006) and Premedline did not yield any relevant reviews or randomised controlled trials of chelation therapy for autism spectrum disorder" (Sinha, Silove, and Williams 2006, p. 756). The president of the American Academy of Pediatrics, Dr. Jay Berkelhamer, told *Dateline:* "The usefulness of chelation therapy in treating autism is nil" (Larson 2006). Dr. Berkelhamer goes on to say, "Chelation therapy is potentially toxic. The chelation materials that are used to remove these metals from the bloodstream can affect the liver and the kidney."

In May 2008, the FDA approved the use of a chelating agent, DMSA, for a controlled, scientific trial of chelation's effectiveness as a treatment for autism. The National Institutes for Mental Health (NIMH), which is the largest funder of autism research in the United States, received pressure from critics for advocating and supporting this line of research. Proponents of the use of chelation saw the approval for this study as a response to parental belief and interest in exploring chelation as a treatment option. As reported in *Nature News,* Dr. Cooper, former president of the

American Academy of Pediatrics said, "that a well-designed study of chelation in children with autism would respond to these parents' deeply held beliefs in the most careful, ethical way." He clarified that "with informed consent, such a study could ensure that the only families to be enrolled would be those already determined to try chelation" (Wadman 2008, p. 259).

Critics in the chelation controversy noted that given there is no evidence to support the mercury poisoning-autism link, there is no evidence to support using a potentially harmful treatment agent. And indeed, chelation can be harmful. In 2005, a 5-year-old boy with autism died following a chelation treatment. While receiving his chelation treatment, the boy, Tariq Nadama, went limp and his mother reported this to the doctor. The medical staff rushed the boy to the hospital, but he died of a heart attack. Following a forensic investigation it was determined that as a result of the chelation process, Tariq's calcium levels dropped, as the chelating agent used in this treatment, EDTA, also binds to calcium. Given the heart's need for calcium in the bloodstream for it to pump and the drastically low calcium levels resulting from chelation, Tariq's heart stopped beating and he died. Two other deaths have been reported as a result of chelation treatment as well (Centers for Disease Control and Prevention 2006).

Based on these reports as well as a research study examining chelation therapy in rodents, the federal government decided to put a halt to pursuing this line of research. In a study conducted to assess the effects of chelation on rodents the authors found that chelation "improves learning, attention, and arousal regulation in lead-exposed rats but produces lasting cognitive impairment in the absence of lead exposure" (Stangle et al. 2007). The findings demonstrated scientifically for the first time that chelation of lead can improve aspects of behavior shown to be impaired in lead poisoning. Importantly the study showed that it is only in the presence of lead poisoning that chelation shows improvement in learning and attention. Two different types of rats were tested in the study: rats with lead exposure and rats without lead exposure. In the rodents not exposed to lead, chelation actually impaired cognition. While the toxic metal in the rodent study was lead and not mercury, the process and chelating agent used in the rodent project was similar to the chelating agent used in children with autism and the agent proposed in the NIMH study.

The proposed applicability of chelation and autism rests on the hypothesis that autism is caused by mercury poisoning. The medical community maintains that there is no evidence to support the theory that autism is caused by mercury poisoning. Given the findings that chelation may actually cause cognitive impairment if it is administered to a patient (as supported by the rodent study) without heavy metal poisoning, opponents of chelation treatment hold that it can have harmful cognitive effects beyond being ineffective and putting the patient at risk for death.

Despite the lack of scientific support for its effectiveness and the risk of significant harm including death, many parents and practitioners have used and continue to use chelation as a form of treatment for autism.

The Gluten-Free, Casein-Free Diet

An additional treatment that has sparked some controversy and debate in the field of autism is the Gluten-Free, Casein-Free diet (GFCF diet). The GFCF diet involves restricting foods containing gluten and casein. Foods containing the protein gluten include wheat, rye, and oats while the protein casein is found in dairy products like milk, cheese, and yogurt. The diet is very difficult to maintain as these proteins need to be eliminated from the diet and that means monitoring the child's intake at home, school, in restaurants, and anywhere else there may be food or other products containing gluten or casein. For example, in addition to food these proteins are found in substances such as Play Doh and glue.

The theoretical rationale for the use of this diet is that in individuals with gastrointestinal problems, such as leaky gut, proteins such as gluten and casein are believed to pass through the permeable membrane of the intestines and into the bloodstream. Once in the bloodstream, these proteins are proposed to cause an immune response and impact functioning of the central nervous system resulting in social withdrawal and psychopathology. This notion was first presented by Dr. F. Curtis Dohan as a possible mechanism for schizophrenia following an experience in the south pacific (Dohan 1966). During his experience in Papua New Guinea and other South Pacific islands, he noted the reduced rate of schizophrenia and postulated the community diet that lacked gluten and casein might play a role. The theory behind the GFCF diet is that through the removal of the proteins that create the toxic peptides absorbed through the leaky gut, neuropathological symptoms can be ameliorated (Seim and Reichelt 1995).

The connection between this diet and autism is based on the observation that increased amounts of opioid peptides based on food proteins have been found in individuals with autism (Reichelt and Knivsberg 2003) and that children with autism have increased rates of gastrointestinal disorders (D'Eufemia et al. 1996). Several studies have demonstrated a greater incidence of gastrointestinal problems in autism, while others have shown no greater incidence than in control populations (Black, Kaye, and Jick 2002; Melmed et al. 2000). Taken as a whole the research in gastrointestinal illness suggests that there is not a general relation between gastrointestinal disorders and autism, but that there may be a connection in a subset of cases (Molloy and Manning-Courtney 2003). Although greater incidence of a "leaky gut" in autism remains under debate, the dietary intervention is based upon this rationale.

Anecdotal reports fuel this argument for the effectiveness of this treatment. The impetus for pursuing GFCF interventions is based upon parental reports of the effectiveness. In a newsletter from the Autism Research Institute, one mother relays her child's encounter with gluten and casein while on the diet. "He was averse to using a glue stick so his teacher rubbed it all over his palm so he could get used to the texture. Within the hour he was screaming violently for the first time all year" (Autism Research Institute 2009, p. 1). Reports such as this one in which parents conclude that behavioral disturbances are the result of exposure to gluten and casein are common in parent support groups and bolster support for GFCF as a treatment for autism.

The experimental studies that have been conducted examining the GFCF diet fail to demonstrate an effectiveness of this treatment in autism and controlled studies are recommended (Millward et al. 2008). There have been only few studies conducted and those that have been have reported findings on small samples and have not controlled for experimental biases. It is difficult to conduct well-designed dietary studies for many reasons. Firstly, it is difficult to maintain these diets because of the widespread use of gluten and casein in so many foods. That makes it difficult as an experimenter to monitor and maintain the diet as an experimental protocol. Secondly, although the diet is in widespread use, in order to conduct a controlled study it would be important for scientists to randomly assign families to either the GFCF diet or nonrestricted diet. This requires recruiting families who have not had prior experience with the diet and families who are willing to either participate in the diet or not, based on random determination. The importance of having a large sample is that this allows for the generalizability of the results. If a study finds that a specific intervention is helpful for a small group of eight or nine children with autism it is difficult to conclude that it will be effective for all children with autism. Thirdly, as mentioned earlier, the concept of blindness is important in scientific studies of treatments, but is hard to implement in dietary studies because it is challenging for parents and experimenters maintaining a specific diet for children to not know what types of food the children are consuming.

In a well-designed treatment study, research participants are tested on a number of variables that the treatment is believed to effect. In autism these variables may include aspects of autism symptomology such as cognitive ability, social ability, language ability, response to transitions, and frequency of repetitive behaviors. Often these abilities are measured by clinical observation and parent report. The assessment of these variables prior to administering the treatment is called the pretest assessment. Then, individuals are randomly assigned to one of at least two interventions. In a GFCF diet intervention, this would mean having half of the children with autism being placed on the diet for a specified period of time while the other half receives a control diet. Following the dietary intervention, the pretest variables would be reassessed. This is called post-testing. If the post-testing reveals an improvement in abilities relative to pretesting in the children receiving the GFCF diet but not in the children receiving the control diet then researchers can conclude that the diet is effective. However, it is essential that the posttesting is conducted by individuals who do not know what intervention the research participant received. This "blindness" is essential to reduce subtle biases that inadvertently affect a clinician's observation of the child or parent report. This "experimenter bias" could then skew the results and indicate a significant improvement in posttest scores relative to pretest scores, when in fact there is no difference.

This type of controlled study with blind raters, large samples, and random assignment has not been conducted on the GFCF diet and autism. As a result, it is not possible to comment on its effectiveness yet. A preliminary study of this type of design has been conducted in a small group of 15 children with autism (Elder et al. 2006). In this well designed study, the diet appeared to not have a significant effect on behavior.

Research is still needed to determine the effectiveness of the intervention. Although existing evidence suggests that the diet is not effective, at least for the majority of children with autism, a review of the scientific literature does not reveal any significant adverse effects (Millward et al. 2008). However, nutritional monitoring would be essential before embarking on a GFCF diet and the implementation of the diet without consideration of the nutritional needs and status of the child could be harmful. It is important to note that many children with autism have restricted food preferences to begin with, which makes implementing the diet and meeting nutritional needs even more difficult. This is especially relevant given that a study published in the *Journal of Autism and Developmental Disorders* found thinner, less dense bones in boys with autism compared to typical peers, which the authors attributed to less exercise, digestive problems, more restricted diets, lack of vitamin D, and reduced intake of casein due to diets in the children with autism (Hediger et al. 2008).

In summary, the effectiveness of the intervention remains under debate. However, several small, well-designed research studies suggest it is ineffective for most children of autism. Clearly more research is needed in this area. While a review of the scientific literature indicates there is limited harm caused by the disorder, the importance of maintaining adequate nutrition is paramount and the time, money, and dedication required to maintain the diet could reduce time and money needed to facilitate treatments that have been shown to be effective.

Conclusion

The controversies that surround interventions in autism stem from the wishes of the autism community (parents, clinicians, teachers, and scientists) to provide effective and efficient treatments. The controversies revolve around treatments that have limited validity as to their efficacy according to scientific examination, but that have strong testimonials from parents. Without a definitive causal mechanism and corresponding intervention pathway, it leaves the door open for debate regarding therapeutic options. That is, options that could be ruled out if the active therapeutic ingredient ran counter to the causal mechanism of the disorder. At the root of many of the controversial treatments in autism is a controversial debate regarding the origin of the disorder. At the root of the chelation debate is the controversy regarding mercury and autism. At the root of the GFCF diet debate is the heated debate about gastrointestinal illness and autism. But there are additional factors that set the scene for these controversies: the cultural context influences both scientific and public ideas about causality of psychiatric disorders as it did in the 1950s and 1960s to support the refrigerator mother theory. The widespread availability of both information and misinformation can mislead and misguide the uninformed observer as happened with secretin. Finally, given the only empirically supported treatment, behavioral intervention, is costly, lengthy, and incredibly time consuming, it is difficult for parents to wait for the slow and meticulous pace of science. The scientific method's value is in the process of peer review, replication, and the careful administration of controlled studies. These all take considerable time. The method for translating scientific findings to clinicians and the public adds additional time and opens the door for miscommunication or communication that lacks the appeal of the testimony of a parent of a child with autism in the same position as the mothers and fathers seeking answers and directions for treatment of their child. Controversy is sure to erupt in these situations.

Even the notion of treating autism itself sparks controversy for some. Organizations have developed and activists have risen to promote the idea that individuals with autism do not need to be "cured" and that treatment is not needed as much as understanding. Aspies for Freedom is one such organization that started in 2004 to speak against abusive treatments and promote awareness of the advantages to having an ASD. On the Aspies for Freedom Web site, it states, "we know that autism is not a disease, and we oppose any attempts to 'cure' someone of an autism spectrum condition, or any attempts to make them 'normal' against their will" (Aspies for Freedom, 2010).

There have been several controversies concerning autism since Leo Kanner first described 11 children with the disorder in 1943. Debates concerning the cause of autism and the appropriate treatment of autism continue today. However, these controversies have not obstructed the forward movement and advancement of our understanding of autism. In many cases, the controversies have spurred on new findings and led to positive changes, such as the development of the first parent run advocacy program in support of parents first vilified as the cause of autism.

Much like Jimmy, the boy with autism who loved Harry Potter, and his family went through a developmental process, so too has the field of autism. Jimmy's parents first noted that something was not quite typical about Jimmy's development when his language developed slowly and he showed less interest in others than they expected. They sought out answers for what caused this from clinicians and through independent research into the available literature. They met with professionals and received a diagnosis of autism. Then they pursued treatment options with the same energy and devotion to their child as they did with identifying what was causing their child's social withdrawal and repetitive behaviors. Throughout this process, they made advances and had setbacks, but always they moved forward for the betterment of Jimmy and their family. So, too, has the field of autism moved forward with advances and setbacks as the field has worked to answer the questions about what caused autism and what should we do about it.

References

American Academy of Pediatrics. 1999. "Joint Statement of the American Academy of Pediatrics (AAP) and the United States Public Health Service (USPHS)" *Pediatrics* 104 (3): 568–69.

Aspies for Freedom. 2010. "Index Page." http://www.aspiesforfreedom.com.

Autism National Committee. 2008. "Autism National Committee (Autcom) Policy and Principles Regarding Facilitated Communication." http://www.autcom.org/articles/PPFC.pdf.

Autism Research Institute. 2009. "Why My Child Is on a Special Diet." http://www.autism.com/families/diet/GFCF_science.pdf.

Bailey, A., A. Bailey, A. Le Couteur, I. Gottesman, P. Bolton, E. Simonoff, E. Yuzda, and M. Rutter, 1995. "Autism as a Strongly Genetic Disorder: Evidence from a British Twin Study." *Psychological Medicine* 25 (1): 63–77.

Bell, C. 1977. *Principles and Applications of Metal Chelation.* Oxford, U.K.: Clarendon Press.

Bernard, S., A. Enayati, L. Redwood, H. Roger, and T. Binstock. 2001. "Autism: A Novel Form of Mercury Poisoning." *Medical Hypotheses* 56 (4): 462–71.

Bettelheim, B. 1967. *The Empty Fortress: Infantile Autism and the Birth of the Self.* New York: The Free Press.

Black, C., J. Kaye, and H. Jick. 2002. "Relation of Childhood Gastro-intestinal Disorders to Autism: Nested Case-control Study Using Data from the U.K. General Practice Research Database." *British Medical Journal* 325 (7361): 419–21.

Boseley, S. 1999. "Parents' Fear Puts Britain at Risk of Rubella Epidemic." *Guardian*, March 19, 1999. http://www.guardian.co.uk/uk/1999/mar/19/sarahboseley.

Bradstreet, J. , D. Geier, J. Kartzinel, J. Adams, and M. Geier. 2003. "A Case-Control Study of Mercury Burden in Children with Autistic Spectrum Disorders." *Journal of American Physicians and Surgeons* 8 (3): 76–79.

Carrey, J. 2009. "The Judgment on Vaccines Is In???" *Huffington Post.* http://www.huffingtonpost.com/jim-carrey/the-judgment-on-vaccines_b_189777.html.

Cedillo v. Secretary of Health and Human Services Case No. 98-916v. 2009. "Decision Statement." United States Court of Federal Claims.

Centers for Disease Control and Prevention. 2006. "Deaths Associated with Hypocalcemia from Chelation Therapy—Texas, Pennsylvania, and Oregon, 2003–2005." *Journal of the American Medical Association* 295 (18): 2131–33.

CNN. 2008. "Vaccine Case Draws New Attention to Autism Debate." *CNNhealth.com,* http://www.cnn.com/2008/health/conditions/03/06/vaccines.autism/index.html#cnnSTCvideo.

Cohen, M. H., and D. M. Eisenberg. 2002. "Potential Physician Malpractice Liability Associated with Complementary and Integrative Medical Therapies." *Annals of Internal Medicine* 136 (8): 596–603.

Dawson, G. 2008. "Statement by Dr. Geri Dawson Chief Science Officer, Autism Speaks." Autism Speaks. http://www.autismspeaks.org/dawson_statement_vaccine_case.php.

Deer, B. 2009. "MMR Doctor Andrew Wakefield Fixed Data on Autism." *Sunday Times,* February 8, 2009.

DeNoon, D. 2008. "Thimerosal Down but Autism Rising: Removal of Mercury from Child Vaccines Fails to Halt Autism Increase." *WebMD Health News.* http://www.webmd.com/brain/autism/news/20090212/vaccine-court-rejects-autism-claims.

Department of Developmental Services. 1999. *Changes in the Population of Persons with Autism and Pervasive Developmental Disorders in California's Developmental Services System: 1987 through 1998.* Sacramento, CA: California Department of Developmental Services.

Derbyshire, D., and C Brahic. 2002. "Scientists Challenge Claims of Steep Rise in Autism." *Telegraph (UK)*, September 6, 2002.

D'Eufemia, P., M. Celli, R. Finocchiaro, L. Pacifico, L. Viozzi, M. Zaccagnini, E. Cardi, and O. Giardini. 1996. "Abnormal Intestinal Permeability in Children with Autism." *Acta Paediatrica* 85 (9): 1076–79.

Dohan, F.C. 1966. "Cereals and Schizophrenia Data and Hypothesis." *Acta Psychiatrica Scandinavica* 42 (2): 125–52.

Edelson, S. 2008. "The Secretin Story: Still a Promising Treatment for Autism." *Autism Research Review International* 22 (2): 3, 6.

Elder, J. H., M. Shankar, J. Shuster, D. Theriaque, S. Burns, and L. Sherrill. 2006. "The Gluten-Free, Casein-Free Diet in Autism: Results of a Preliminary Double Blind Clinical Trial." *Journal of Autism and Developmental Disorders* 36 (3): 413–20.

Filipek, P.A., P.J. Accardo, G.T. Baranek, E.H. Cook Jr., G. Dawson, B. Gordon, J.S. Gravel, et al. 1999. "The Screening and Diagnosis of Autistic Spectrum Disorders." *Journal of Autism and Developmental Disorders* 29 (6): 439–84.

Folstein, S., and M. Rutter. 1977. "Infantile Autism: A Genetic Study of 21 Twin Pairs." *Journal of Child Psychology and Psychiatry* 18 (4): 297–321.

Freitag, C.M. 2007. "The Genetics of Autistic Disorders and Its Clinical Relevance: A Review of the Literature." *Molecular Psychiatry* 12 (1): 2–22.

Generation Rescue. 2009. "Index Page." http://www.generationrescue.org.

Geschwind, D.H. 2009. "Advances in Autism." *Annual Review of Medicine* 60:367–80.

Grinker, R. 2007. *Unstrange Minds: Remapping the World of Autism*. New York: Basic Books.

Harris, G. 2008. "Measles Cases Grow in Number and Officials Blame Parents' Fear of Autism." *New York Times*, August 21, 2008.

Hazelhurst v. Secretary of Health and Human Services Case No. 03-654v. 2009. "Decision Statement." United States Court of Federal Claims.

Hediger, M.L., L.J. England, C.A. Molloy, K.F. Yu, P. Manning-Courtney, and J.L. Mills. 2008. "Reduced Bone Cortical Thickness in Boys with Autism or Autism Spectrum Disorder." *Journal of Autism and Developmental Disorders* 38 (5): 848–56.

Horton, R. 2004. "The Lessons of MMR." *Lancet* 363 (9411): 747–49.

Horvath, K., G. Stefanatos, K.N. Sokolski, R. Wachtel, L. Nabors, and J.T. Tildon. 1998. "Improved Social and Language Skills after Secretin

Administration in Patients with Autistic Spectrum Disorders." *Journal of the Association for Academic Minority Physicians* 9 (1): 9–15.

Institute of Medicine. 2004. "Immunization Safety Review: Vaccines and Autism." Washington, D.C.: National Academies Press.

Kanner, L. 1943. "Autistic Disturbances of Affective Contact." *Nervous Child* 2:217–50.

Kirby, D. 2005. *Evidence of Harm: Mercury in Vaccines and the Autism Epidemic: A Medical Controversy.* New York: St. Martin's Press.

Larson, J. 2006. "The Unorthodox Practice of Chelation." *Dateline,* edited by NBC News. http://www.msnbc.msn.com/id/13102473/.

Lilienfeld, S., and H. Arkowitz. 2007. "Is There Really an Autism Epidemic?" *Scientific American* 17: 58–61.

Lister, S. 2009. "Sleep Rise in Measles Blamed on MMR Scare." *Times Online,* February 6, 2009. http://www.timesonline.co.uk/tol/life_and_style/health/child_health/article5674974.ece.

McCarthy, J., and J. Carrey. 2008. "Jenny McCarthy: My Son's Recovery from Autism." *CNN,* http://www.cnn.com/2008/US/04/02/mccarthy.autsimtreatment/index.html.

McLellan, D. 1999. "Andrew Awakes." *Ladies Home Journal* 116: 162–66.

Melmed, R., C. Schneider, R. Fabes, J. Phillips, and K. Reichelt. 2000. "Metabolic Markers and Gastrointestinal Symptoms in Children with Autism and Related Disorders." *Journal of Pediatric Gastroenterology and Nutrition* 3: S31–S32.

Millward, C., M. Ferriter, S. Calver, and G. Connell-Jones. 2008. "Gluten- and Casein-Free Diets for Autistic Spectrum Disorder (Review)." *Cochrane Database of Systematic Reviews,* Issue 2: 1–14.

Molloy, C. A., and P. Manning-Courtney. 2003. "Prevalence of Chronic Gastrointestinal Symptoms in Children with Autism and Autistic Spectrum Disorders." *Autism* 7 (2): 165–71.

Morrice, P. 2005. "What Caused the Autism Epidemic?" *New York Times,* April 17, 2005.

Murch, S., A. Anthony, D. Casson, M. Malik, M. Berelowitz, A. Dhillon, M. Thomson, A. Valentine, S. Davies, and J. Walker-Smith. 2004. "Retraction of an Interpretation." *Lancet* 363 (9411): 750.

Offit, P. 2008. *Autism's False Prophets: Bad Science, Risky Medicine, and the Search for a Cure.* New York City: Columbia University Press.

Pauley, J. 1998. "Breaking the Silence." *Dateline NBC,* October 7, 1998.

Reichelt, K. L., and A. M. Knivsberg. 2003. "Can the Pathophysiology of Autism Be Explained by the Nature of the Discovered Urine Peptides?" *Nutritional Neuroscience* 6 (1): 19–28.

Research Units on Pediatric Psychopharmacology Autism Network. 2002. "Risperidone in Children with Autism and Serious Behavioral Problems." *New England Journal of Medicine* 347 (5): 314–21.

Rimland, B. 1964. *Infantile Autism.* New York: Appleton-Century-Crafts.

Rogers, L. 2004. "Scientists Desert MMR Maverick." *Sunday Times (UK),* March 7, 2004.

Sandler, A. D., K. A. Sutton, J. DeWeese, M. A. Girardi, V. Sheppard, and J. W. Bodfish. 1999. "Lack of Benefit of a Single Dose of Synthetic Human Secretin in the Treatment of Autism and Pervasive Developmental Disorder." *New England Journal of Medicine* 341 (24): 1801–6.

Schechter, R., and J. K. Grether. 2008. "Continuing Increases in Autism Reported to California's Developmental Services System: Mercury in Retrograde." *Archives of General Psychiatry* 65 (1): 19–24.

Schreibman, L. 2005. *The Science and Fiction of Autism.* Cambridge, MA: Harvard University Press.

Seim, A. R., and K. L. Reichelt. 1995. "An Enzyme/Brain-Barrier Theory of Psychiatric Pathogenesis: Unifying Observations on Phenylketonuria, Autism, Schizophrenia and Postpartum Psychosis." *Medical Hypotheses* 45 (5): 498–502.

Shapiro, H., ed. 1998. "Secretin Discussion." In *Pediatric Development and Behavior.* Developmental-Behavioral Pediatrics Online Community. http://www.dbpeds.org.

Shattuck, P. T., M. Durkin, M. Maenner, C. Newschaffer, D. S. Mandell, L. Wiggins, L. C. Lee, et al. 2009. "Timing of Identification among Children with an Autism Spectrum Disorder: Findings from a Population-Based Surveillance Study." *Journal of the American Academy of Child and Adolescent Psychiatry* 48 (5): 474–83.

Sinha, Y., N. Silove, and K. Williams. 2006. "Chelation Therapy and Autism." *British Medical Journal* 333 (7571): 756.

Snyder v. Secretary of Health and Human Services Case No. 01-162v. 2009. "Decision Statement." United States Court of Federal Claims.

Stangle, D. E., D. R. Smith, S. A. Beaudin, M. S. Strawderman, D. A. Levitsky, and B. J. Strupp. 2007. "Succimer Chelation Improves Learning, Attention, and Arousal Regulation in Lead-Exposed Rats but Produces Lasting Cognitive Impairment in the Absence of Lead Exposure." *Environmental Health Perspectives* 115 (2): 201–9.

Sturmey, P. 2005. "Secretin Is an Ineffective Treatment for Pervasive Developmental Disabilities: A Review of 15 Double-Blind Randomized Controlled Trials." *Research in Developmental Disabilities* 26 (1): 87–97.

Taylor, Z. 2007. "Autism Epidemic Being Ignored." *Daily Telegraph (AU)*, May 12, 2007.

Wadman, M. 2008. "Autism Study Panned by Critics." *Nature* 453 (7202): 259.

Wakefield, A. J. 2009. "In His Desperation, Deer Gets It Wrong Again." *Age of Autism: Daily Web Newspaper of the Autism Epidemic*, http://www.rescuepost.com/files/deer-response.pdf.

Wallis, C. 2007. "Is the Autism Epidemic a Myth?" *Time*, January 12, 2007.

Wallis, C. 2008. "Case Study: Autism and Vaccines." *Time.com*, March 10, 2008. http://www.time.com/time/health/article/0,8599,1721109,00.html.

Wegner, D., V. Fuller, and B. Sparrow. 2003. "Clever Hands: Uncontrolled Intelligence in Facilitated Communication." *Journal of Personality and Social Psychology* 85 (1): 5–19.

Wiggins, L. D., J. Baio, and C. Rice. 2006. "Examination of the Time between First Evaluation and First Autism Spectrum Diagnosis in a Population-Based Sample." *Journal of Developmental and Behavioral Pediatrics* 27 (2, Suppl.): S79–S87.

Wiggins, L., C. Rice, and J. Baio. 2009. "Developmental Regression in Children with an Autism Spectrum Disorder Identified by a Population-Based Surveillance System." *Autism* 13 (4): 357–74.

3

Worldwide and Cultural Perspectives in ASD

Introduction

Individuals with Autism Spectrum Disorder (ASD) represent a heterogeneous population and come from a large variety of cultural backgrounds. Research has suggested that, aside from a well-documented differential male-to-female sex ratio of 4:1, the diagnosis occurs approximately equally across ethnicities and cultures (Bertrand et al. 2001; Department of Health and Human Services 2002). Additionally, the behavioral manifestation of the disorder appears to be similar across cultures and countries. No studies to date have reported significant ethnic differences in symptom presentation (Mandell and Novak 2005). However, much variation exists both across and within cultures in terms of the acceptance of an ASD diagnosis, appraisal of its etiology, views on sources of family support, and availability and acceptability of treatment options.

Culture is a complex concept with many different in depth meanings. In this chapter, culture will be defined as a set of perceptions, beliefs, values and/or behaviors that are passed on from generation to generation via a shared context, such as a common language, history, or geographic location (Hays 2005). Cultural influence is a powerful aspect of an individual's development of identity, kinship, and views about the world. Culture is also commonly confused with other related terms. For instance, it is often used interchangeably with *race* and *ethnicity*. However, culture does not imply a shared biology, as has often been the case with many definitions of the latter two terms.

The definition of race has been a controversial topic for some time. The concept of race originated from European scientists in order to categorize people into genetically related groups based on geography and certain physical characteristics, such as skin color and facial features (Hays 2005). Unfortunately, this proved to serve as a basis for hierarchically classifying individuals in society based purely on physical features. Additionally, it failed to take into account the huge variation of physical characteristics observed within racial groups. For example, the range of skin tones in persons of African descent typically varies from very dark to very light and there is often overlap between Anglo Americans with darker skin and African Americans of lighter skin. In recent years, some racial categories (e.g., African American) have come to also imply a sense of heritage and shared social history in addition to (or, in fact, instead of) physical characteristics.

Hays (2005, p. 12) defines ethnicity as a shared ancestry involving communal values and customs that are "generally understood to involve some shared biological heritage, [but] its more important aspects in terms of individuals and group identify are those that are socially constructed (e.g., beliefs, norms, behavior, and institutions)."

Research examining cultural factors in ASD is slim and has not received abundant financial or research attention. A number of reasons exist for the lack of priority given to this aspect of ASD. The frequently disabling and pervasive nature of the disorder may prevent cultural factors from being adequately considered due to the multitude of other issues (e.g., diagnostic process, treatment planning, and associated medical symptoms) that families, providers, and researchers are forced to manage. Additionally, well-replicated findings in the past three decades have revealed the disorder's strong roots in biological processes, including genetic factors and neurological functions. Therefore, cultural environment *may* be assumed to play no role in the disorder because biology appears to be very influential in its development. However, although actual symptoms of biologically based diseases may be comparable across cultures, how the symptoms are described, interpreted, and accepted into society varies widely. Consider cancer as an example. Actual physical symptoms of cancer are generally the same whether a person has the disease in Uruguay, Ghana, or China. But how the patient and his/her family within these various cultures understands, labels, and responds to the disease may be incredibly different. While more developed countries may quickly label the group of symptoms as "cancer" or a linguistic equivalent and treat with chemotherapy, others may view the symptoms as spiritual punishment and treat with herbal remedies or religious interventions. Views and knowledge about ASD are variable both across countries and in cultures and ethnicities within countries such as the United States.

Macro cultural factors (i.e., factors occurring at the dominant culture level affecting the majority of people in that society) can play a large role in the level of functioning and outcome of an individual with ASD. Such factors include availability of services, cultural acceptance of the disorder, and existence of national and/or state-funded treatment options. In addition to larger macro cultural factors, individual response and acceptance of the diagnosis varies at a micro cultural level within families. Prior to the first ASD genetic findings in 1977 (Folstein and Rutter 1977), a commonly held position was that family culture, particularly cold, aloof parenting style, was responsible for the development of ASD in an individual. This Refrigerator Mother Theory, which has been discussed at length in previous chapters, has been disproved as a causal factor in ASD. However, although maternal behavior and parenting style are clearly not related to the *occurrence* of ASD in their child, parental response to receiving the diagnosis, family views about ASD, and chosen next steps make an impact on the child's prognosis. Therefore, in addition to a consideration of larger cultural factors potentially affecting the prognosis of a child, family-specific factors are influential as well.

Prevalence Rates

ASD is a disorder that knows no cultural boundaries and appears to occur at approximately equal rates across countries, ethnicities within a country, and social classes. Additionally, rates of diagnosis are increasing at comparable percentages across these various cultures. Although controversy has existed, and continues to exist, about differential occurrence in, for instance, families within upper socioeconomic status (SES) and families immigrating from other countries, overall scientific evidence continues to point toward an equal distribution of ASD across all cultures.

Epidemiological Studies

The field of epidemiology studies the distribution of disease in human populations and influential factors in the presentation of the disorder. Important measures of disease within the field include "incidence rates," which refers to the number of new cases occurring over a period of time, and "prevalence rates" signifying the proportion of subjects who, at a given point in time, have a disease. The vast majority of epidemiological studies of ASD have been cross-sectional in nature and report prevalence rates. Therefore, these studies will be included in the discussion.

Dr. Eric Fombonne, a prominent epidemiologist and ASD expert, conducted a review of epidemiological studies of ASD in 2005. Using surveys from a range of countries, he found international median prevalence rates of ASD to be 13/10,000 for autistic disorder, 21/10,000 for Pervasive Developmental Disorders—Not Otherwise Specified (PDD-NOS), and 2.6/10,000 for Asperger's Disorder (Fombonne 2005). Some reported estimates range from 22/10,000 in the United Kingdom (Chakrabarti and Fombonne 2005), to 7.2/10,000 in Denmark (Madsen et al. 2002), to 13.2/10,000 in Iceland (Magnusson and Saemundsen 2001), to 66/10,000 in the United States (Centers for Disease Control and Prevention 2007). In his review, Fombonne (2005) found that prevalence rates were related to sample size such that studies with fewer participants reported higher prevalence rates. Additionally, there was a large degree of variability in samples, even within the same country due to different methodologies used in the epidemiological studies. How the diagnosis is made and ability to capture more subtle diagnoses such as Asperger's Disorder and PDD-NOS, varies across countries as well. Fombonne (2005, p. 289) suggests that "epidemiological surveys of ASD each possess unique design features, which could account almost entirely for between-studies variations in rates," implying that the true prevalence rates are likely comparable across countries.

Difficulty in obtaining prevalence rates in some countries is common due to a variety of factors, such as increased childhood mortality, poverty, and health issues. Many cultures may not recognize ASD as a disorder or may group these individuals under another category. A lack of consistent health records in some countries makes data on the prevalence of ASD or associated risk factors unavailable. Additionally, as will be discussed in subsequent sections of this chapter, cultural beliefs and practices often impact recognition and integration of ASD into society. Therefore, some individuals with ASD may be missed and true estimates impacted in epidemiological studies.

Immigrant Status

There has been some debate concerning increased rates of ASD diagnosis among individuals whose parents have immigrant status (e.g., Gillberg et al. 1987; Wing 1980). More recently, increased prevalence of ASD in Somali immigrants has been reported in Sweden (Barnevik-Olsson, Gillberg, and Fernell 2008) as well as more informal reports in the United States from the state of Minnesota (see Minnesota's Department of Health fact sheet, http://www.health.state.mn.us/ommh/projects/autism/reportfs090331.pdf). However, Fombonne states that evidence for increased ASD rates in individuals with immigrant status is inconclusive given the variability of results across studies and relatively small sample sizes found in many surveys. Large-scale epidemiological estimates do not support the finding of increased prevalence rates in immigrant families. For example, Croen and colleagues (2002) reported on prevalence rates of "full syndrome ASD" (which excluded diagnoses of Asperger's Disorder, PDD-NOS, Childhood Disintegrative Disorder, and Rett's Disorder) in the state of California in birth cohorts over the course of a seven-year period. Prevalence rates were approximately equal across ethnic and racial groups, including families with immigrant status. Fombonne (2007) summarizes his and many other expert's view by stating that, "the hypothesis of an association between immigrant status or race and ASD, therefore, remains largely unsupported by the empirical results" (p. 60).

Social Class

In Leo Kanner's original work describing individuals with ASD, he observed "There is one other very interesting common denominator in the backgrounds of these children. *They all come of highly intelligent families*" (1943, p. 248). Although Dr. Kanner's statement refers to the parents' intelligence, he did not actually conduct cognitive/intelligence testing with them. Instead, he went on to describe their educational background and various professions, such as physician, lawyers, and professors. Articles in the 1960s and 1970s from the United Kingdom, Denmark, Japan, and the United States also found elevated rates of ASD in families with higher levels of education who were of upper SES (e.g., Lotter 1966; Treffert 1970).

However, acquisition of participants in earlier epidemiological studies partially depended on families' access to services. Since families of higher SES can access services more readily than those of lower SES, it is likely that the association between ASD diagnosis and higher SES is an artifact of attainment bias in the studies (Fombonne 2007). More recent estimates with more rigorous and comprehensive methodology find no association with parent education or SES and ASD diagnosis (e.g., Croen et al. 2002). This suggests that ASD affects individuals of all socioeconomic backgrounds at an equal rate.

Cultural Influences in Mental Disorders

Cultural factors influencing perception, treatment options, and response to diagnosis have received little research attention in the field of ASD relative to other areas. The majority of ASD studies do not include culture as a significant variable nor do they attempt to include individuals from diverse cultural groups (Mary 1990). However, inferences about cultural impacts in ASD can be drawn from research within other fields and/or disorders related to ASD. ASD is considered to be a developmental disability, classified under the category of mental disorders.

Within the United States and elsewhere, cultural sensitivity in diagnosis and treatment of mental disorders has been an increasing area of emphasis due to significant concerns about the disparities in access to and availability of mental health care for racial and ethnic minorities (Department of Health and Human Services 2001). For example, African American children in the United States and their families are less likely to seek out and use mental health services compared to other groups (Cooper-Patrick et al. 1999; Diala et al. 2000). Furthermore, once African American families are in mental health treatment, they more often report having negative experiences (Diala et al. 2000) and remain in therapy for a shorter period of time than Anglo Americans (Bui and Takeuchi 1992; Cuffe et al. 1995). Many Asian Americans experience shame and disgrace when acknowledging that emotional problems have brought them to seek mental health services instead of handling the problems themselves, within the family environment (Sue and Sue 2008). Such cultural factors often discourage Asian Americans from pursuing mental health treatment at all.

With respect to children, Lau et al. (2004) found that Asian American and African American parents less often agreed with teacher concerns that their children's challenging classroom behaviors were a result of an underlying disorder (instead of a variation of normal behavior) than Anglo American parents. Therefore, some families from nondominant cultures may be less likely to interpret their child's behaviors as problematic. If they do not perceive the child's behaviors to be interfering with functioning, then they will, naturally, less often seek treatment or services for said behaviors. Parents of children from low-income and minority groups may more often be less educated, lack access to information, and experience greater exclusion from educational services (Bennett 1988; Harry 1992). These factors put them at risk for less knowledge about and access to services.

The use of cultural sensitivity in the diagnosis and treatment of mental disorders has been shown to be effective in helping to establish and maintain positive clinical relationships. Cultural sensitivity is defined by O'Donohue (2005) as knowledge of which cultures a client/family belong, comfort with some basic facts about social rules and customs within these cultures, and knowing when it is appropriate to apply such rules. Consultation with a member of the client/family's within a clinician's profession is also recommended to ensure culturally sensitive care.

Cultural Factors Related to Developmental Disabilities

In addition to existing discrepancies in the use of mental health services, differences also exist in how developmental disabilities specifically are diagnosed and treated among ethnic groups. Family adaptation to their child's condition, views on its etiology, and the impact of religion and social support on family functioning can vary widely.

Family Adaptation

Much is known about family adaptation to raising a child with developmental disabilities (Seligman 1999) and, as discussed in Dyches, Wilder, and Obiakor (2001), ethnicity is beginning to be considered as a significant factor in a family's adjustment to children in the family with developmental disabilities. Parallels can be drawn between general developmental delays and ASD, but caution should be used because of stressors that differentiate ASD from other developmental disabilities. Modal cultural views and responses will be described, but specific family adaptation will, of course, vary depending on the particular child's strengths and challenges and individual family response.

Dyches, Wilder, and Obiakor (2001) describe the Resiliency Model of Family Stress, Adjustment, and Adaptation ("Resiliency Model"), which was originally developed as a means to explore how ethnicity and culture come into play in the adaptation of families with low income to life stressors. This model was first presented by McCubbin et al. (1998) and emphasizes ethnic and culture factors as influential in the development of new patterns of functioning and reestablishment of balance within a family following a family stressor. A stressor does not necessarily have to be perceived as negative. Graduating from high school, changing jobs, and, perhaps, receiving a diagnosis of a developmental disability in a youngster can be interpreted as positive stressful life events.

Family Appraisal

Family appraisal or determination of the gravity of the stressor is a component of the adjustment phase of the Resiliency Model. In this case, the stressor of the diagnosis of a developmental disability may be appraised differently across cultures. As described in Dyches, Wilder, and Obiakor (2001), a negative appraisal often arises when the medical model is applied—that "something is wrong" or "diseased" in individuals with developmental disabilities that needs to be "fixed." The application of this medical model often occurs with Anglo Americans living in the United States. Even the English word *disability* reflects the medical model, focusing on abilities that are "not" there. Negative appraisals about the origin of developmental disabilities also occur in cultures such as Mojaves (Green, Sack, and Pambrum 1981) and Navajos (Connors and Donnellan 1998) where it is believed that a child's disabilities stem from the parents' transgressions. Shame is often associated with diagnoses of developmental disabilities and mental health disorders in modal Asian cultures (Sue and Sue 2008). Stigma about disabilities is also a concern in Middle Eastern countries, such as the United Arab Emirates. Feelings of shame about the diagnosis and related challenges are common in parents, particularly fathers. Yet, mothers in one study appeared to be resolved to provide the best care possible for their children (Crabtree 2007).

Native Hawaiian and Native American cultures tend to focus more on the child's abilities that *are* present and his/her "normal" behavior (whatever degree is present) rather than *dis*abilities and unusual behaviors (McCubbin, Thompson et al. 1998). Many low-income African American families are less likely to consider their child with a disability to be a significant burden as compared to Anglo Americans and report experiencing positive gains and personal growth from their child with a disability. Reports suggest that as the child with the disability reaches adulthood, they would prefer to keep him/her at home rather than obtaining outward help through a group home or more structured residential care (Heller and Factor 1988; McCallion, Janicki, and Grant-Griffin 1997; Valentine, McDermott, and Anderson 1998). Yet another study with African American families reported that families feared the stigma of a diagnosis (Pruchno, Patrick, and Burant 1997).

Appraisal can vary within cultures as well. Latino women from a younger generation have been reported to view a child with a disability as a blessing and an opportunity to rise to the challenge of bringing up a special child whereas older generations in the Latino culture may believe the child to be a punishment for wrongdoing (Skinner et al. 1999).

Religion

Religious beliefs are also an important cultural factor to consider as influential in a family's adjustment to a developmental disability such as ASD. In modal American culture, the consideration of religion and/or spirituality in the care of a child with special needs represents a divergence from the typical practice of separating church from state. However, religion can and often does play an important role in the coping process of families with a child with a disability. Religion may serve as both a source spiritual support and informal support through religious institutions (Tarakeshwar and Pargament 2001). It also influences child-rearing practices and helps to define the role of the help-giver and the nature of "help" itself.

One study compared religious perspectives among Latino families who had children with developmental disabilities. Those families whose religious perspectives were likely to encourage the belief that having a child with a developmental disability is a punishment from God for sins were impacted more negatively than those families whose religious perception was that the child was special and "chosen" by God (Gannotti et al. 2001). Religions associated with modal African American culture emphasize acceptance and importance of all children and may be more likely to encourage a positive appraisal of ASD (Rogers-Dulan and Blacher 1995). A female caregiver from an African American family who had a child with a disability commented, "They [the people at church] treat her like there wasn't nothing wrong with her. They treat her like us. Like regular—like they would treat others" (Terhune 2005, p. 21).

However, views on religion can vary within a cultural group. A number of low-income African American women (e.g., mothers, aunts, etc.) who were primary caregivers for family members with disabilities were interviewed about their experience raising an individual with a disability (Terhune 2005). The influence of "God" came up in every interview in relation to the women's experience of raising a child with a disability. However, the particular type of influence God had on the caregivers varied.

A subgroup of women in this study, those with a more "secular discourse" as labeled by the author, viewed God as a distant, judgmental figure who had no direct influence on the occurrence of positive events in their lives (Terhune 2005). They tended to rely on services from professionals such as educational and treatment providers to support the child with special needs. In contrast, those women who reported having a more intimate relationship with God viewed Him as benevolent, caring, and actively involved in their day-to-day lives. One mother stated, "What my faith has done for me is to help me to know that that light that I keep saying I see is there. And it is going to come forth. I don't believe she [my child with a disability] was put into our lives just by happenstance" (Terhune 2005, p. 21). These women tended to view the challenges associated with raising the child as manageable and more often focused on the "blessings" in their lives, such as good respite care and a positive school classroom. In summary, for some individuals within a culture, having a strong faith can be beneficial in terms of support to manage the routine stress in life. Others, however, may not experience religious faith in the same way and may rely instead on professionals as the primary care providers and source of support.

Social Support

According to Dyches, Wilder, and Obiakor (2001), another component of the adjustment phase of the Resiliency Model that is relevant to adjustment to disabilities is the use of social support, including family, friends, neighbors, and community supports such as church and parent support groups. Type and level of social support varies widely across cultures. Many cultures, such as modal Native Hawaiian (McCubbin, Thompson et al. 1998), Filipino (McCubbin, Thompson et al. 1998), Latino (Blacher et al. 1997), and African American (Pruchno, Patrick, and Burant 1997) cultures emphasize a broader cooperation among family members (both immediate and extended) and members of the community to care for an individual in need. Caregiver stress is often perceived to be lower in these groups, perhaps due to the shared provision of care for the child with disabilities.

An approach for provision of services that may be particularly relevant for groups who rely heavily upon broader social supports is called Family-Centered Practice. Family-Centered Practice involves prioritizing the choices of the family to drive the delivery of services, rather than delivery based on preferences of the system (and associated professionals) and child-specific needs. It recognizes that the family is the constant in the child's life while the service systems and personnel within those systems fluctuate. Family-Centered Practice is more flexible than more traditional forms of service delivery and encourages constant reflection upon the best treatment options possible for the particular family. It may, for example, involve offering choices to families and empowering the family to help decide the best course of action for their child. Interaction with and inclusion of professionals, caregivers, and community support (e.g., close friends, members of their church, and support group leaders) in treatment planning is essential. Many families report that informal social support through parents of other children with disabilities, close friends and family, and other community supports is more influential than professional support. Therefore, helping the family to activate informal social supports is considered to be an important component of Family-Centered Practice.

One randomized, controlled trial examined outcomes and follow-up support for high risk infants during the first year of life (Affleck et al. 1989). One arm of the study offered weekly in-home visits from professionals while another arm of the study involved treatment as usual, without regularly scheduled in-home visits. Results suggested that for families in the in-home visit group who had an informal social support network in place, weekly visits were often viewed as a burden and poor use of their time. For families with low levels of informal social support, these visits were perceived more positively. Affleck and colleagues' (1989) results can be extended to the field ASD such that for families of children with ASD who have in tact informal support, less professional services may be warranted. Making those families without much social support aware of supports available in their community, such as parent-led support groups for families of children with ASD, may be helpful. Overall, Family-Centered Practice involving an assessment of the level of social support available to families would be beneficial to providing the most effective support for the individual family.

Cognitive Testing

Although access to and use of mental health providers is lower in racial and ethnic minorities, studies have found that ethnic minority groups are overrepresented in public special education programs (Harry et al. 1995). In order to qualify for special education services in school, cognitive and other related types of testing are conducted to determine eligibility for school-provided services. Much controversy exists about the appropriateness and applicability of standardized cognitive testing for all ethnic groups. Such aspects of testing as the nature of assessment tools and the evaluation environment have been questioned regarding their cultural sensitivity. Children of particular ethnic minority statuses consistently score lower on cognitive assessments compared to Anglo American children (Sattler and Dumont 2004). For instance, in the normative sample used in the *Wechsler Intelligence Scale for Children, Fourth Edition* (*WISC-IV*, Wechsler 2003), Anglo American children as a whole had a full scale IQ score that was 11.5 points higher than that of African American children and 10 points higher than Latino children—almost a one standard deviation difference in scores. On the other hand, Asian American children scored 3.5 points higher than Anglo American children on the *WISC-IV* (Sattler and Dumont 2004).

The differential scores have often been attributed to the disproportionate percentage of these minority groups in the lower income brackets compared to Anglo Americans (Sattler 2001). Although most minority families in the United States are not living in poverty, there is an overrepresentation of some groups living below the poverty level, particularly Latinos, African Americans, and Native Americans (21.2%, 24.7%, and 25.3%, respectively, compared to 10.5% of whites and 10.6% of Asian Americans; U.S. Census Bureau 2008). For children living in poverty, there is often increased stress due to parents holding multiple jobs, less access to educational opportunities such as tutoring, and decreased occurrence of preeducational activities such as reading. Additionally, exposure to toxic substances such as lead-based paint and living in areas with poor air quality are common in poverty-stricken households. Scores on cognitive tests may be impacted by the negative effects associated with living in a lower income household and/or one that is impacted by poverty (Turkheimer et al. 2003).

Although this is one potential causal factor for decreased cognitive scores, another is that the cognitive tests may be culturally and linguistically biased. A recent study found that bilingual children with autism of ethnic minority status scored lower on language assessments compared to Anglo American children, unrelated to SES (Leadbitter and Hudry 2009). Differences may arise from the faulty assumption that the dominant culture values apply for all cultures and these assumptions become embedded in these assessments. For instance, one verbal subtest of a commonly used cognitive assessment in the United States requires knowledge of the U.S. government and familiarity with normative social behavior. A child who, for instance, recently immigrated to the United States and who had limited awareness of the governmental process and little exposure to the social norms of the country would have difficulty answering these questions "correctly." Thus, scores may be lowered not due to decreased intellectual abilities, but as a result of limited exposure to the cultural norms of the dominant society.

Language barriers also exist in assessments, which places some cultural and ethnic groups at risk for negatively impacted scores. Incorrect responses may be attributed to decreased fluency with the test language rather than actual ability level. To address potential language barriers, it is ideal to conduct diagnostic and/or cognitive assessments in the child's native language, if the clinician is fluent. If not, then using independent interpreters who are knowledgeable in the family's native culture, rather than family or friends, can be helpful. This serves to decrease potential bias in interpretation and maximize child response (Harry et al. 1995).

A child's familiarity with the examiner appears to improve cognitive testing scores for all children (Fuchs and Fuchs 1989). However, it seems to be particularly influential for children of minority status and/or from low-income families. African American and Latino children scored approximately 11 IQ points higher with a familiar as compared to an unfamiliar examiner. Familiarity with the examiner did not alter scores for Anglo American children as a whole. Similarly, for children from low-SES families (regardless of race), scores were more improved with a familiar examiner compared to changes in score for children from middle- to upper-SES families (Fuchs and Fuchs 1989).

These arguments that have been raised describing potential bias in tests have helped to improve the cultural sensitivity of cognitive testing by, for example, encouraging test-makers to expand the normative sample from which standardized tests are drawn to better reflect the demographics of the region. Additionally, test items now undergo more scrutiny to minimize cultural bias (Sattler 2001). However, standardized tests continue to need modifications to become more culturally sensitive.

Cultural Factors and ASDs

ASD is often perceived to be a particularly stressful developmental disability (Randall and Parker 1999). Unlike some other developmental disabilities such as Down Syndrome, ASD cannot be detected in utero or at birth and does not have any associated physical characteristics that are observable from the outside. From a parent's perspective, there are not outward signs that something is different about their child. As infants who eventually go on to receive an ASD diagnosis grow older, parents often only gradually realize that their child is not developing normally and not achieving the developmental milestones at the same rate (if at all) as their nieces, nephews, or friends' children. These differences are generally not recognized until well into infancy or toddler years because social and language skills do not begin to mature in typically developing infants until late infancy and/or toddlerhood. So, for a significant amount of time in the child's life, differences are not pronounced, if detectable at all, and parents (naturally) assume that their child is normal and "perfect."

Therefore, in addition to the pervasiveness of eventual challenges, families often grieve the loss of their "perfect" child once a diagnosis is given (Dyches, Wilder, and Obiakor 2001). This complex process can be particularly devastating for families whose children experience a significant regression in skills after developing normally for some time. Therefore, although research examining cultural factors associated with general developmental disabilities provides insight into ASD, there may be additional and important considerations related specifically to having a child with ASD.

ASD Symptoms and Diagnosis

Cultural variation exists in social behaviors. What is considered "normal" social conduct in one culture may be atypical in another. Since ASD is at its core a disorder of reciprocal social interactions, it is crucial to consider cultural norms when determining whether a behavior is considered deviant. Certain symptoms of ASD may in fact be acceptable in particular cultures. For instance, modal Asian culture considers making direct eye contact with authorities to be a sign of disrespect. Children are taught to avoid eye contact with adults out of respect (Lian 1996; Sue and Sue 2008). In a typical ASD assessment, an adult who is likely to be considered an authority figure attempts to engage a child in social interaction and notes concern if the child does not make eye contact. In fact, impairment in nonverbal social behaviors such as eye contact is one of the diagnostic criteria for all ASDs. By extension, a child raised in modal Asian culture may avoid eye contact not because they have ASD, but because they are following the social norms of their culture.

Peer relationships are another area in which cultural influences may be confounded. Some families who live in remote or rural areas or who do not have other children in the family may have limited exposure and practice with peer interactions. Therefore, challenges in peer relationships may not be due to fundamental challenges in social skills, but rather to a lack of experience with same-aged peers. Therefore, clinicians must act with cultural sensitivity when considering whether or not ASD is an appropriate diagnosis.

Diagnostic Tools

The Autism Diagnostic Observation Schedule (ADOS; Lord et al. 1999) and Autism Diagnostic Interview (ADI; Lord, Rutter, and Le Couteur 1994) are considered to be gold standard assessment tools in diagnosing ASD (Filipek et al. 1999). These tools have made significant improvements in standardizing the assessment of ASD and allow for better comparison across research studies. However, these measures were not designed to capture cultural variables.

Although the ADOS has been translated into 12 languages (Danish, Dutch, Finnish, French, German, Hungarian, Icelandic, Italian, Korean, Norwegian, Spanish, and Swedish), the impact of translation without modifications for potential cultural confounds has not been thoroughly assessed. Caution must be considered as to the applicability and appropriateness of using these instruments in cultures other than those in which they were created.

Countries outside of the United States

There is limited research examining cultural views about ASD specifically in other countries. This may partly be because many cultures and languages do not have a word or label for autism or ASD. For instance, Native Hawaiian and Native American languages use longer descriptions of behaviors associated with ASD to describe the condition rather than a single word (Connors and Donnellan 1998). Additionally, some Asian languages do not have a word for ASD (Dobson et al. 2001) while others use a label that does not accurately reflect the disorder. For instance, *autism* translates to "lonely disease" in China, which, as many Chinese parents complain, does not capture the true nature of the disorder (McCabe 2007). Other languages have simply adapted the English word (e.g., *autismo* in Spanish and Italian) and, according to Wilder and colleagues (2004), possibly the values that go along with it.

The few studies examining cultural and family response to ASD in non-Western cultures will be described. Although a thorough literature review was conducted, it is possible that some sources may have been missed. A recent study examining mother's experience of raising a child with ASD in an Ultraorthodox Jewish community in Israel suggests that ASD may be associated with mystical forces in this culture (Shaked and Bilu 2006). The authors state that this community believes that "autistic children have sublime souls with direct access to the otherworldly" (Shaked and Bilu 2006, p. 20). Facilitated communication, described in detail in Chapter 2 and repeatedly found by controlled studies to be an ineffective intervention, continues to be used in the Ultraorthodox Jewish community in Israel. Facilitated communication involves the use of adult support of a child's hand while he/she types on a keyboard to communicate and is viewed in this community in Israel as a way for children with autism to "impart hidden knowledge from heaven" (Shaked and Bilu 2006, p. 20).

Chinese culture tends to view ASD in a more negative light. Special education was first introduced in China in the 1970s, but parents continue to be rarely involved in the educational planning of their children. As discussed, stigma exists about mental illness in Chinese culture (e.g., Tsang et al. 2003), and families often feel shamed about having a child with a disability—believing it occurred as punishment for parent, particular maternal, behavior. The continued existence of societal pressures for conformity in China allows little room for the acceptance of individual differences, such as child disabilities. Furthermore, in more rural parts of the country, the diagnosis of ASD is relatively unknown to both professionals and parents and children with ASD are often turned away from services.

Forty-three caregivers of a child with ASD were interviewed about their experiences raising their child in China (McCabe 2007). Despite a societal disapproval of ASD, parents appear to continue to want the best for their children. Most families in the study devoted an incredible amount of time and resources to their child. A father explained, "When a person realizes their child, at age 3, age 5, realizes that their child is not normal, they will begin to ask everywhere, look everywhere. This is because for Chinese people, we do everything for our children, children are the hope of parents . . . it was extremely hard on us, but what can you do? It's for our child" (McCabe 2007, p. 47). However, all families relayed their fear that their children would be discriminated against based on their disability and the family judged for the child's ASD due to the traditional Chinese belief that the child's behavior and success directly reflects upon the parents. One mother described, "It's as if, when other people run into this thing [having a child with a disability], maybe people where we're from will laugh, point at you behind your back" (McCabe 2007, p. 43). Families were also concerned about their child receiving proper care and services. The stigma of a diagnosis of a disability may discourage families from seeking out an evaluation and reporting a diagnosis to the school. In addition to modal Chinese culture, some South Asian families reported hesitation in referring their child for services because of the stigma associated with the diagnosis and possible negative impact on arranged marriages, particularly for girls (Raghavan, Weisner, and Patel 1999).

Roy Grinker, a professor of Anthropology at George Washington University in Washington, D.C., is a father of a daughter with severe autism who traveled around the world interviewing parents of children with ASD. He published some of his experiences in a book entitled *Unstrange Minds: Remapping the World of Autism.*

In his visit to South Africa, Grinker (2007) describes the commonly held belief by Europeans who colonized Africa that Africans were assumed to be "too primitive" to suffer from mental illnesses because of their lack of exposure to stresses associated with life in industrialized societies. When Africans did show signs of mental illness, they were kept in what essentially were prisons rather than hospitals. This unfounded belief is gradually changing and there are now psychiatric hospitals and treatment facilities available to treat mental disorders, but Africans are naturally suspicious of them because of this history. Grinker (2007) shares one story of a Zulu child from Africa with ASD who experienced a severe regression in skills. The boys' grandparents recommended that he see a traditional Zulu healer, a *nygana*, to determine the cause of the boy's strange movements and sudden lack of eye contact. The nygana viewed his onset of challenges as punishment from the family's ancestors for wrongdoing and believed that a demon spirit had possessed him. Although his parents eventually took him to a psychiatrist in South Africa, many traditional healing methods were attempted before this last, and more successful, treatment effort took place.

In India, autism was only recognized as a disorder separate from intellectual disability (previously known as *mental retardation*) in 1999. However, many children continue to be mislabeled as having intellectual disability or are considered to be "mad" (*paagol* in Hindu). Few professionals can actually diagnose ASD, and religious healers are often first consulted to help cure children. Medical providers who have heard of ASD will often prescribe medications or vitamins rather than recommending behavioral interventions that have been shown to be effective, although this has been changing in recent years (Grinker 2007). In his book, Grinker (2007) relays the story of the mother of a boy with ASD in India who, after going to great lengths to get him a diagnosis from one of the few psychiatrists in New Delhi, could not enroll him in an autism treatment or educational program because they did not exist. So, she decided to open her own school for children with ASD.

An American psychologist, Tamara Daley, eventually met up and worked with this mother to increase the awareness about ASD in India. Part of Daley's work involved studying Indian parent's recognition and interpretation of ASD symptoms.

Daley (2004) found that Indian parents were more likely to notice social difficulties as compared to parents from the United

States who were more likely to detect general developmental delays or regression in language skills (Coonrod and Stone 2004). In fact, language delays are not considered by some Indian parents and professionals to be a core feature of ASD because of the often-held belief that boys acquire speech later than girls (Daley and Sigman 2002). Daley hypothesizes that these differences may be due to the fact that Indian culture values social conformity while culture in the United States is more focused on language development.

Racial and Ethnic Groups within the United States

As discussed in the introduction of this chapter, the use and meaning of the term *race* has been historically controversial. However, demographic information continues to be collected using race as a variable in both clinical and research settings. Therefore, for the purposes of discussing research collected using this methodology, racial groups will be included in the discussion. However, caution should be used when applying sets of beliefs and behaviors to such groups. A study of Medicaid-eligible children with ASD in Philadelphia county found that Anglo American children receive a diagnosis about one and a half years, on average, earlier than African American children and two and a half years earlier than Latino children (Mandell et al. 2002). Additionally, African American children spent more time in treatment before receiving the diagnosis of ASD. A follow-up study found that African American children ultimately diagnosed with ASD were nearly three times more likely than Anglo American children to be diagnosed with another disorder first such as conduct or adjustment disorder (Mandell et al. 2007). One possible interpretation put forth is that African American parents might have been more likely to emphasize their children's disruptive behavior during the assessment rather than social oddities. Other explanations are that these racial differences in diagnosis may be attributable to general prejudices held by the clinician, specific stereotypes about health-related behaviors, and statistical discrimination in which the clinician can have different expectations about the probability of ASD occurring in children of different ethnicities (Balsa, McGuire, and Meredith 2005).

In the United States, the Individuals with Disabilities Education Act (IDEA) requires an annual report of all children who receive educational services under this law. Reports generally include the number and percentage of children served under various disability categories, including ASD. Dyches, Wilder, and Obiakor (2001) reviewed the U.S. Department of Education's 2001 IDEA report and found that the percentage of children served under the category of ASD differed based on the race of the child. Students identified as African American or Asian/Pacific Islander were served under the category of ASD at twice the rate of those who were American Indian/Alaskan or Hispanic. Unlike true epidemiological studies, these percentages do not indicate the actual diagnosis of children. A number of factors may influence these discrepant statistics, including actual differences in the prevalence of ASD across races (although this has not been supported by research), how individuals are categorized ethnically, and/or reluctance of families within some cultures in labeling their child with ASD in the school system (Dyches, Wilder, and Obiakor 2001).

Given that norms for social interactions, general behaviors (e.g., tantrums), and communication skills are culturally based, the context in which these "symptoms" occur needs to be carefully considered by school professionals and other treatment providers. It is possible that children identified under the "autism" category are misclassified.

Acquisition of Cultural Knowledge

Cultural influences on family's perception and adjustment to the diagnosis have been discussed at length. A related area is how children with ASD perceive cultural cues and acquire knowledge about their culture. Loth and Gómez (2006) state that "cultural knowledge is seen as a prism through which all experiences are filtered. It influences how we perceive and interpret the world, it endows us with knowledge and expectation of what kinds of things happen in different events, which social behavior is "good" or "bad," permitted, allowed, or obligated" (p. 157). How children come to know and engage in social interaction is a cultural experience and varies significantly depending on which culture and family they are raised. We begin with an understanding of how typically developing children learn about their culture. Much of social learning originates from imitation (i.e., copying an observed action). Imitation interacts with the ability to take another's perspective. This cognitive ability is called *theory of mind*.

Typically developing infants are born with the seemingly innate ability to imitate (Meltzoff and Moore 1977)—beginning with facial expressions and moving on to more complex social behaviors such as gestures and play skills. The development of language also involves the use of social understanding. Word learning involves the directing of infants' attention to the object of focus through non-verbal means such as pointing and eye gaze (e.g., Tomasello 1992). For example, looking toward a cup, holding it up, and pointing to it while repeatedly saying "cup" is more effective than simply saying "cup" without these extra social cues. Following a person's point or eye gaze to an object of interest is posited to be a precursor to more advanced forms of theory of mind as it involves the basic insight that a social partner has a different perspective of the world. The use of someone else's cues to direct one's attention to an object or event of interest is called *joint attention*. Loth and Gómez (2006) suggest that these skills are essential in the acquisition of skills *through* others and that much of our learning, particularly early in life, occurs through these means. Studies have suggested that learning about one's culture, including social norms and rules, is acquired through these basic processes that are then expanded upon as children grow older (e.g., Bloom 2004; Clément, Koenig, and Harris 2004).

Children with ASD have been shown to have deficits in a variety of different kinds of imitation (see Rogers 1999 for a review; e.g., Williams, Whiten, and Singh 2004) and joint attention skills (e.g., Dawson et al. 1998). For those individuals who do have intact imitation skills, the way in which they imitate may be unusual (Loth and Gómez 2006). Therefore, these necessary building blocks in beginning to understand and acquire cultural knowledge are absent or delayed in children with ASD. This puts them at risk for missing cultural knowledge generally learned *through* another person by imitation and theory of mind. In fact, deficits in knowledge of social norms and cultural rules have been documented in individuals with ASD (Baron-Cohen et al. 1999).

The Culture of Autism

Although not traditionally considered a culture in and of itself, higher functioning individuals with ASD have advocated that "autism" be considered and treated as its own cultural group. Supporters of this view wish to be recognized as a group having values, beliefs, and behaviors that are to be respected. Therefore, some views held by members of this group warrant acknowledgement in a discussion about cultural influences in ASD.

By and large, the professional and scientific community promotes identification and treatment of ASD symptoms. However, there is a rising group of supporters called the Autism Rights Movement who instead encourage and embrace the "neurodiversity" of individuals and resist finding a cure for ASD. They encourage the acceptance of individuals with ASD in the community as they are, without studying them or trying to fix them. Many Internet Web sites and groups exist in support of this stance, including the Autistic Self Advocacy Network and the Autism Network International. Another such group is called Aspies for Freedom, and their mission statement is as follows, "We have the view that aspergers and autism are not negative, and are not always a disability. . . . We know that autism is not a disease, and we oppose any attempts to 'cure' someone of an autism spectrum condition, or any attempts to make them 'normal' against their will. We are part of building the autism culture. We aim to strengthen autism rights, oppose all forms of discrimination against aspies and auties, and work to bring the community together both online and offline" (http://www.aspiesforfreedom.com/).

The culture of the pro-autism movement is to accept ASD as a variation in functioning as opposed to a mental disorder. The movement adheres to the belief that ASDs are indeed genetically based and should be considered as part of the natural expression of the human genome, not genetic mutations. Their hope is to be accepted as a minority group in need of representation, rather than a disabling condition in need of repair.

Treatment

Access to Services

Research has shown that behavioral treatment is the only intervention that has been empirically demonstrated to be effective for children with ASD (National Research Council 2001). However, well-trained treatment providers are often associated with large universities or hospitals in metropolitan areas. There is limited access to qualified ASD treatment providers in rural areas and in many countries whose acceptance and understanding of ASD is low. For instance, in Taiwan, suburban and rural children with ASD tended to receive the diagnosis at an older age and to have a longer diagnosis process as compared with urban children (Chen et al. 2008). Additionally, behavioral interventions are very costly to implement and they are generally not covered through public funding. These factors together place families who live in such areas or who cannot afford treatment at a disadvantage for obtaining the most effective interventions for their children, if they are able to obtain services at all (Thomas et al. 2007).

Disparities in access to and use of services of individuals living in rural areas and racial and ethnic minorities are common for all children both with and without special health care needs (e.g., Newacheck, Hung, and Wright 2002; Stevens and Shi 2003). In ASD, lower rates of diagnosis and access to treatment for Latino, African American, and socio-economically deprived families have been noted (Liptak et al. 2008). Thomas et al. (2007), among others, found that racial and ethnic minority families are less likely to use such services as a case manager, psychologist, and developmental pediatrician. More limited use of services by racial and ethnic minorities may be partially explained by a lack of appropriate outreach and cultural competency of providers (e.g., Lau et al. 2004) as well as a general mistrust of the system due to institutionalized discrimination (Schnittker 2003). An additional explanation is that these families are more likely to rely upon extended family members and friends rather than meet with professionals who do not know their child personally and are part of a larger institution of which families are unfamiliar (Terhune 2005).

Cultural Influences in Treatment Choice

Cultural values influence how a family chooses a treatment and responds to various treatments. In the general field of mental health, treatment decisions are often made based on a family's belief about the etiology of the diagnosis. As discussed, understanding of etiology varies across cultures. African American, Asian American, and Latino families may be less likely to view their child's symptoms as related to a health condition and therefore may be less likely to seek care through traditional medical systems and instead may pursue alternative therapies, such as diet changes and supplemental vitamins (Bussing, Schoenberg, and Perwien 1998; Yeh et al. 2004). Cultural decisions about treatment choices in ASD was examined in one small study and found that Latino children diagnosed with ASD were six times more likely to be treated using nontraditional strategies than children of other ethnicities (Levy et al. 2003). Parents in North Carolina who completed a higher level of education were found to use more and different kinds of therapy services (e.g., Picture Exchange Communication System and therapeutic horseback riding) as compared to families with fewer years of completed education (Thomas et al. 2007).

Treatments that are commonly used in the United States to improve ASD symptoms have rarely been researched to examine their effectiveness in other countries. A recent exception to this is the Treatment and Education of Autistic and related Communication-handicapped Children (TEACCH), developed by Eric Schopler. TEACCH provides a structured teaching environment and includes parents as cotherapists to aid in the treatment and education of children with ASD. It has recently received positive research support for its effectiveness in improving ASD symptoms in a group of children in China (Tsang et al. 2007). Comparison groups are now necessary to determine its effectiveness compared to other treatments in China. In traditional Chinese medicine, ASD is viewed as any other illness would be—as an imbalance in the energy of yin and yang. ASD is considered to be a "yin" disorder, involving social withdrawal and inwardness, with recommended traditional treatments such as acupuncture and Chinese herbs. However, more recent use of applied behavior analysis and sensory integration training, and now TEACCH are growing increasingly common (Clark and Zhou 2005).

Focus of Treatment

Varying cultural perspectives can also affect how intervention goals are prioritized in an ASD treatment plan. For instance, modal culture for Anglo Americans includes placing a high value on individualism whereas other cultures have a more collectivist orientation, prioritizing the group over the individual. It may be more important for some families to focus on behaviors in their child that facilitate family and community activities rather than individual competence and autonomy. This could potentially clash with behavioral treatments often aimed at fostering independence and teaching self-help skills such as making clear requests and performing tasks independently. For example, an often-held Western goal for long-term outcome of individuals with disabilities, including those with ASD, is to hold a steady job in their adult life. However, those providing treatment to individuals with should be aware that family expectations of families from a non-Western background might hold different expectations of their child in terms of long-term goals.

Differences in child-rearing practices and cultural values have implications for therapists and educators working with parents of children with ASD and are important for both treatment developers and providers to consider when designing and implementing a treatment plan. For instance, child-rearing practices of Mexican American mothers tend to focus more on teaching politeness and obeying authority figures (e.g., parents and teachers), whereas with Anglo American mothers more often value self-directed learning and independent thinking (Rodriguez and Olswang 2003).

An examination of differences in views on the expression of emotion further elucidates the impact of culture on treatment goals. Individuals with ASD often have difficulty recognizing and expressing emotion; thus, many treatments are geared toward helping individuals express their emotions. However, many Asian cultures value private over public displays of emotion and discourage outward emotional displays. A treatment attempting to elicit outward emotional expression may contradict the values of these cultures. Additionally, parents are often asked to be an active member of the treatment team and implement interventions at home and other settings for their child. But the role that parents take in treatment and the expected role of teachers and other clinicians varies across cultures—some cultures may expect therapists and educators to be the main providers and assume that parents do not need to be involved.

The style of teaching used with individuals with ASD may also be an area where compromise is necessary. For instance, the general educational environment in many Asian societies involves systematic and repeated practice of a newly acquired skill in a structured learning setting. This could potentially clash with an ASD treatment provider who uses a more naturalistic style of teaching, involving following the child leads and offering choices through play (as in the Denver Model; Sally Rogers). Treatments providers may need to adapt their style of service in order to collaborate effectively with families.

Treatment/Educational Recommendations

Dyches, Wilder, and Obiakor (2001) recommend several strategies for working with individuals with ASD in an educational and treatment setting. Primarily, examining and being comfortable acknowledging one's own personal prejudices are part of an essential groundwork for providing the best education and care of children from multicultural backgrounds. Possible prejudice may exist against groups based on such factors as religion, income, gender, race, ethnicity, personal appearance, and disability. This can be an emotionally taxing and difficult realization for care providers and yet crucial to determine whether these views are interfering with the effectiveness of intervention. Although a seemingly obvious objective, viewing each child with ASD in a positive light and as capable of growth, regardless of ability level or cultural background, is central to helping them meet their treatment goals. Provider and teacher expectations of children with disabilities, including ASD, are also influential in treatment. Expectations may vary for children of different backgrounds, whether consciously acknowledged or not. Studies have found that when teachers have high expectations of children, they tend to meet or exceed those expectations (Lucas, Henze, and Donato 1990).

Language is also an important consideration. There is an overrepresentation of children from bilingual backgrounds in special education. This implies that professionals conducting assessments to determine eligibility for special education may have difficulty distinguishing fluency and comfort with dominant language from a true disability. If a student who is not fluent in the dominant language is identified for special education, then special education providers need to collaborate with the teacher responsible for instructing students who do not speak the nondominant language to help implement educational and behavioral interventions (Dyches, Wilder, and Obiakor 2001). Speech and language therapy may also be warranted and should often be considered as part of an overall treatment plan or an Individualized Education Program (IEP). If available, bilingual educational and treatment providers are also recommended to help ensure better understanding of material for children. Peer mentors can also be helpful in providing acculturation experiences and social skills training in the dominant culture, should that be recommended for the individual student.

In terms of a broader educational curriculum, it has been noted that multicultural students in general education are negatively impacted by the lack of exposure in the classroom to history, events, and educational experiences outside of the dominant culture (Dyches et al. 2004). Therefore, efforts can and should be made to incorporate such curricula into education to encourage feelings of belonging in students from a multicultural background, including those students with ASD.

Conclusion

Epidemiological studies suggest that ASD occurs at approximately equal rates across cultures, including countries, races, ethnicities, and income levels. However, cultural differences exist in terms of interpretation of symptoms, views about its etiology, possible stigma associated with the diagnosis, and treatments employed to address symptoms. ASD is primarily a disorder of social interactions. However, social behaviors and rules are culturally derived and what is considered abnormal in one culture may be socially appropriate in another. Clinicians making diagnoses must consider the child's behavior within the context of their own culture when conducting an evaluation and deciding if ASD is an appropriate diagnosis.

Research examining cultural views about ASD specifically is slim. However, conclusions about such issues can be drawn from work on cultural factors relating to general mental health and developmental disabilities. For instance, some cultures have a positive appraisal of developmental disabilities and encourage the belief that children with a developmental disability are special or even chosen by God. They may also view the experience of raising the child as an opportunity for parents to challenge themselves and grow personally. Still others believe that parents/families who have a child with disabilities are being punished for parental or familial transgressions. For many cultures, there continues to be stigma associated with acknowledging that the child is different. This often discourages families from informing providers about the child's diagnosis or from seeking help at all. However, with increased awareness about ASD and other developmental disabilities, these stigmas are beginning to dissipate.

Given the multitude of views about the cause of developmental disabilities such as ASD, it is not surprising that a variety of treatment approaches and styles exist as well. Beliefs about the etiology of an individual's difficulties and treatment choices often occur in concert. More effective behavioral interventions are relatively unknown in some countries and traditional medicinal or religious healers are often the first choice of treatment for ASD. Others emphasize treatment goals of increased independence while some cultures may value group cohesion and cooperation over self-sufficiency in treatment planning. Therefore, those working with individuals with ASD must be sensitive to such cultural differences when offering treatment choices to families and implementing treatment programs.

References

Affleck, Glenn, Howard Tennen, Jonelle Rowe, and Beth Roscher. 1989. "Effects of Formal Support on Mothers' Adaptation to the Hospital-to-Home Transition of High-risk Infants: The Benefits and Costs of Helping. *Child Development* 60 (2): 488–501.

Balsa, Ana I., Thomas G. McGuire, and Lisa S. Meredith. 2005. "Testing for Statistical Discrimination in Health Care." *Health Services Research* 40 (1): 227–52.

Barnevik-Olsson, Martina, Christopher Gillberg, and Elisabeth Fernell. 2008. "Prevalence of Autism in Children Born to Somali Parents Living in Sweden: A Brief Report." *Developmental Medicine & Child Neurology* 50 (8): 598–601.

Baron-Cohen, Simon, Michelle O'Riordan, Valerie Stone, Rosie Jones, and Kate Plaisted. 1999. "Recognition of Faux Pas by Normally Developing Children with Asperger Syndrome or High-functioning Autism." *Journal of Autism and Developmental Disorders* 29 (5): 407–18.

Bennett, Adrian T. 1988. "Gateways to Powerlessness: Incorporating Hispanic Deaf Children and Families into Formal Schooling." *Disability, Handicap & Society* 3 (2): 119–51.

Bertrand, Jacquelyn, Audrey Mars, Coleen Boyle, Frank Bove, Marshalyn Yeargin-Allsopp, and Pierre Decoufle. 2001. "Prevalence of Autism in a United States Population: The Brick Township, New Jersey, Investigation." *Pediatrics* 108 (5): 1155–61.

Blacher, Jan, Steven Lopez, Johanna Shapiro, and Judith Fusco. 1997. "Contributions to Depression in Latina Mothers with and without Children with Retardation: Implications for Caregiving." *Family Relations* 46 (4): 325–34.

Bloom, Paul. 2004. *Descartes' Baby: How the Science of Child Development Explains What Makes Us Human*. New York: Basic Books.

Bui, Khanh-van T., and David T. Takeuchi. 1992. "Ethnic Minority Adolescents and the Use of Community Mental Health Care Services. *American Journal of Community Psychology* 20 (4): 403–17.

Bussing, Regina, Nancy E. Schoenberg, and Amy R. Perwien. 1998. "Knowledge and Information about ADHD: Evidence of Cultural

Differences among African-American and White Parents." *Social Science & Medicine* 46 (7): 919–28.

Centers for Disease Control and Prevention. 2007. "Prevalence of Autism Spectrum Disorders—Autism and Developmental Disabilities Monitoring Network, 14 Sites, United States, 2002." *MMWR Surveillance Summaries* 56 (1): 12–28.

Chakrabarti, Suniti, and Eric Fombonne. 2005. "Pervasive Developmental Disorders in Preschool Children: Confirmation of High Prevalence." *The American Journal of Psychiatry* 162 (6): 1133–41.

Chen, Chuan-Yu, Chieh-Yu Liu, Wen-Chuan Su, Su-Ling Huang, and Keh-Ming Lin. 2008. "Urbanicity-related Variation in Help-seeking and Services Utilization among Preschool-age Children with Autism in Taiwan." *Journal of Autism and Developmental Disorders* 38 (3): 489–97.

Clark, Elaine, and Zheng Zhou. 2005. "Autism in China: From Acupuncture to Applied Behavior Analysis." *Psychology in the Schools* 42 (3): 285–95.

Clément, Fabrice, Melissa Koenig, and Paul Harris. 2004. "The Ontogenesis of Trust." *Mind & Language* 19 (4): 360–79.

Connors, Jeanne L., and Anne M. Donnellan. 1998. "Walk in Beauty: Western Perspectives on Disability and Navajo Family/Cultural Resilience." In *Resiliency in Native American and Immigrant Families,* ed. H. I. McCubbin, E. A. Thompson, A. I. Thompson, and J. E. Fromer, 159–82,. Thousand Oaks, CA: Sage Publications.

Coonrod, E. E., and W. L. Stone. 2004. "Early Concerns of Parents of Children with Autistic and Nonautistic Disorders." *Infants and Young Children* 17 (3): 258–68.

Cooper-Patrick, Lisa, Joseph J. Gallo, Neil R. Powe, Donald S. Steinwachs, William W. Eaton, and Daniel E. Ford. 1999. "Mental Health Service Utilization by African Americans and Whites: The Baltimore Epidemiologic Catchment Area Follow-Up." *Medical Care* 37 (10): 1034–45.

Crabtree, Sara Ashencaen. 2007. "Maternal Perceptions of Care-giving of Children with Developmental Disabilities in the United Arab Emirates." *Journal of Applied Research in Intellectual Disabilities* 20 (3): 247–55.

Croen, Lisa A., Judith K. Grether, Jenny Hoogstrate, and Steve Selvin. 2002. "The Changing Prevalence of Autism in California." *Journal of Autism and Developmental Disorders* 32 (3): 207–15.

Cuffe, Steven, Jennifer Waller, Michael Cuccaro, Andres Pumariega, and Carol Garrison. 1995. "Race and Gender Differences in the Treatment of Psychiatric Disorders in Young Adolescents." *Journal of the American Academy of Child and Adolescent Psychiatry* 34 (11): 1536–43.

Daley, Tamara C. 2004. "From Symptom Recognition to Diagnosis: Children with Autism in Urban India." *Social Science & Medicine* 58 (7): 1323–35.

Daley, Tamara C., and Marian D. Sigman. 2002. "Diagnostic Conceptualization of Autism Among Indian Psychiatrists, Psychologists, and Pediatricians." *Journal of Autism and Developmental Disorders* 32 (1): 13–23.

Dawson, Geraldine, Andrew N. Meltzoff, Julie Osterling, Julie Rinaldi, and Emily Brown. 1998. "Children with Autism Fail to Orient to Naturally Occurring Social Stimuli." *Journal of Autism and Developmental Disorders* 28 (6): 479–85.

Department of Health and Human Services. 2001. *Executive Summary—Mental Health: Culture, Race, and Ethnicity. Supplement to Mental Health: A Report of the Surgeon General.* Washington, D.C.: Department of Health and Human Services.

Department of Health and Human Services. 2002. *Report to Congress on Autism.* Washington, D.C.: National Institute of Mental Health, National Institute of Health, and Department of Health and Human Services.

Diala, Chamberlain, Carles Muntaner, Christine Walrath, Kim J. Nickerson, Thomas A. LaVeist, and Philip J. Leaf. 2000. "Racial Differences in Attitudes Toward Professional Mental Health Care and in the Use of Services." *American Journal of Orthopsychiatry* 70 (4): 455–64.

Dobson, Susan, Shripati Upadhyaya, Jeanie McNeil, Shoba Venkateswaran, and Debra Gilderdale. 2001. "Developing an Information Pack for the Asian Carers of People with Autism Spectrum Disorders." *International Journal of Language & Communication Disorders* 36:216–21.

Dyches, Tina Taylor, Lynn K. Wilder, and Festus E. Obiakor. 2001. "Autism: Multicultural Perspectives." In *Autistic Spectrum Disorders: Educational and Clinical Interventions,* ed. T. Wahlberg, F. Obiakor, S. Burkhardt, and A. F. Rotatori, 151–77,. Oxford, England: Elsevier Science Ltd.

Dyches, Tina Taylor, Lynn K. Wilder, Richard R. Sudweeks, Festus E. Obiakor, and Bob Algozzine. 2004. "Multicultural Issues in Autism." *Journal of Autism and Developmental Disorders* 34 (2): 211–22.

Filipek, Pauline A., Pasquale J. Accardo, Grace T. Baranek, Edwin H. Cook Jr., Geraldine Dawson, Barry Gordon, Judith S. Gravel, et al. 1999. "The Screening and Diagnosis of Autistic Spectrum Disorders." *Journal of Autism and Developmental Disorders* 29 (6): 439–84.

Folstein, Susan, and Michael Rutter. 1977. "Infantile Autism: A Genetic Study of 21 Twin Pairs." *Journal of Child Psychology and Psychiatry* 18 (4): 297–321.

Fombonne, Eric. 2005. "The Changing Epidemiology of Autism." *Journal of Applied Research in Intellectual Disabilities* 18 (4): 281–94.

Fombonne, Eric. 2007. "Epidemiological Surveys of Pervasive Developmental Disorders." In *Autism and Pervasive Developmental Disorders (2nd ed.)*, ed. F. R. Volkmarpp. 33–68. New York: Cambridge University Press.

Fuchs, Douglas, and Lynn S. Fuchs. 1989. "Effects of Examiner Familiarity on Black, Caucasian, and Hispanic Children: A Meta-analysis." *Exceptional Children* 55 (4): 303–8.

Gannotti, Mary E., W Penn Handwerker, Nora Ellen Groce, and Cynthia Cruz. 2001. "Sociocultural Influences on Disability Status in Puerto Rican Children." *Physical Therapy* 81 (9): 1512–23.

Gillberg, Christopher, Suzanne Steffenburg, Birgitta Börjesson, and Lena Andersson. 1987. "Infantile Autism in Children of Immigrant Parents: A Population-based Study from Göteborg, Sweden." *British Journal of Psychiatry* 150:856–58.

Green, Ben E., William H. Sack, and Audra Pambrum. 1981. "A Review of Child Psychiatric Epidemiology with Special Reference to American Indian and Alaska Native children." *White Cloud Journal of American Indian/Alaska Native Mental Health* 2 (2): 22–36.

Grinker, Roy Richard. 2007. *Unstrange Minds: Remapping the World of Autism*. New York: Basic Books.

Harry, Beth. 1992. "An Ethnographic Study of Cross-cultural Communication with Puerto Rican-American Families in the Special Education System." *American Educational Research Journal* 29 (3): 471–94.

Harry, Beth, Marquita Grenot-Scheyer, Marsha Smith-Lewis, and Hyun-Sook Park. 1995. "Developing Culturally Inclusive Services for Individuals with Severe Disabilities." *Journal of the Association for Persons with Severe Handicaps* 20 (2): 99–109.

Hays, Pamela. 2005. *Addressing Cultural Complexities in Practice: A Framework for Clinicians and Counselors*. Washington, D.C.: American Psychological Association.

Heller, Tamar, and Alan Factor. 1988. "Permanency Planning Among Black and White Family Caregivers of Older Adults with Mental Retardation." *Mental Retardation* 26 (4): 203–8.

Kanner, Leo. 1943. "Autistic Disturbances of Affective contact." *Nervous Child* 2:217–50.

Lau, Anna S., Ann F. Garland, May Yeh, Kristen M. McCabe, Patricia A. Wood, and Richard L. Hough. 2004. "Race/Ethnicity and Inter-Informant Agreement in Assessing Adolescent Psychopathology." *Journal of Emotional and Behavioral Disorders* 12 (3): 145–56.

Leadbitter, K., and K. Hudry. 2009. "Does Bilingualism Affect Language Development in Autism?" Poster presented at the Annual International Meeting for Autism Research, Chicago.

Levy, Susan E., David S. Mandell, Stephanie Merhar, Richard F. Ittenbach, and Jennifer A. Pinto-Martin. 2003. "Use of Complementary and Alternative Medicine among Children Recently Diagnosed with Autistic Spectrum Disorder." *Journal of Developmental and Behavioral Pediatrics* 24 (6): 418 23.

Lian, Ming-Gong John. 1996. "Teaching Asian American Children." In *Teaching Students with Moderate/Severe Disabilities, Including Autism: Strategies for Second Language Learners in Inclusive Settings (2nd ed.),* ed. E. Durán, pp. 239–53. Springfield, IL: Charles C. Thomas, Publisher.

Liptak, Gregory S., Lauren B. Benzoni, Daniel W. Mruzek, Karen W. Nolan, Melissa A. Thingvoll, Christine M. Wade, and G. Edgar Fryer. 2008. "Disparities in Diagnosis and Access to Health Services for Children with Autism: Data from the National Survey of Children's Health." *Journal of Developmental and Behavioral Pediatrics* 29 (3): 152–60.

Lord, C., M. Rutter, P. C. DiLavore, and S. Risi. 1999. *Autism Diagnostic Observation Schedule—WPS (ADOS-WPS).* Los Angeles: Western Psychological Services.

Lord, C., M. Rutter, and A. Le Couteur. 1994. "Autism Diagnostic Interview-Revised: A Revised Version of a Diagnostic Interview for Caregivers of Individuals with Possible Pervasive Developmental Disorders." *Journal of Autism and Developmental Disorders* 24 (5): 659–85.

Loth, Eva, and Juan Carlos Gómez. 2006. "Imitation, Theory of Mind, and Cultural Knowledge: Perspectives from Typical Development and Autism." In *Imitation and the Social Mind: Autism and Typical Development,* ed. S. J. Rogers and J. H. G. Williams, 157–97. New York: Guilford Press.

Lotter, Victor. 1966. "Epidemiology of Autistic Conditions in Young Children: I. Prevalence." *Social Psychiatry* 1:124–37.

Lucas, Tamara, Rosemary Henze, and Ruben Donato. 1990. "Promoting the Success of Latino Language-Minority Students: An Exploratory Study of Six High Schools." *Harvard Educational Review* 60 (3): 315–40.

Madsen, Kreesten Meldgaard, Anders Hviid, Mogens Vestergaard, Diana Schendel, Jan Wohlfahrt, Poul Thorsen, Jørn Olsen, and Mads Melbye. 2002. "A Population-based Study of Measles, Mumps, and Rubella Vaccination and Autism." *The New England Journal of Medicine* 347 (19): 1477–82.

Magnusson, Pall, and Evald Saemundsen. 2001. "Prevalence of Autism in Iceland." *Journal of Autism and Developmental Disorders* 31 (2): 153–63.

Mandell, David S., Richard F. Ittenbach, Susan E. Levy, and Jennifer A. Pinto-Martin. 2007. "Disparities in Diagnoses Received Prior to a Diagnosis of Autism Spectrum Disorder." *Journal of Autism and Developmental Disorders* 37 (9): 1795–802.

Mandell, David S., John Listerud, Susan E. Levy, and Jennifer A. Pinto-Martin. 2002. "Race Differences in the Age at Diagnosis among Medicaid-eligible Children with Autism." *Journal of the American Academy of Child & Adolescent Psychiatry* 41 (12): 1447–53.

Mandell, David S., and Maytali Novak. 2005. "The Role of Culture in Families' Treatment Decisions for Children with Autism Spectrum Disorders." *Mental Retardation and Developmental Disabilities Research Reviews* 11 (2): 110–15.

Mary, Nancy L. 1990. "Reactions of Black, Hispanic, and White Mothers to Having a Child with Handicaps." *Mental Retardation* 28 (1): 1–5.

McCabe, Helen. 2007. "Parent Advocacy in the Face of Adversity: Autism and Families in the People's Republic of China." *Focus on Autism and Other Developmental Disabilities* 22 (1): 39–50.

McCallion, Philip, Matthew Janicki, and Lucinda Grant-Griffin. 1997. "Exploring the Impact of Culture and Acculturation on Older Families Caregiving for Persons with Developmental Disabilities." *Family Relations* 46 (4): 347–57.

McCubbin, Hamilton I., Marilyn A. McCubbin, Anne I. Thompson, and Elizabeth A. Thompson. 1998. "Resiliency in Ethnic Families: A Conceptual Model for Predicting Family Adjustment and Adaptation." In *Resiliency in Native American and immigrant families*, ed. H. I. McCubbin, E. A. Thompson, A. I. Thompson, and J. E. Fromer, 3–48. Thousand Oaks, CA: Sage Publications.

McCubbin, Hamilton I., Elizabeth A. Thompson, Anne I. Thompson, and Julie E. Fromer. 1998. *Resiliency in Native American and Immigrant Families*. Thousand Oaks, CA: Sage Publications.

Meltzoff, Andrew N., and M. Keith Moore. 1977. "Imitation of Facial and Manual Gestures by Human Neonates." *Science* 198 (4312): 75–78.

National Research Council, Division of Behavioral and Social Sciences Education. 2001. *Educating Children with Autism*. Washington, D.C.: National Academy Press.

Newacheck, Paul W., Yun-Yi Hung, and Kara K. Wright. 2002. "Racial and Ethnic Disparities in Access to Care for Children with Special Health Care Needs." *Ambulatory Pediatrics* 2 (4): 247–54.

O'Donohue, William T. 2005. "Cultural Sensitivity: A Critical Examination." In *Destructive Trends in Mental Health: The Well-intentioned Path to Harm,* ed. R. H. Wright and N. A. Cummings, 29–44 . New York: Routledge.

Pruchno, Rachel, Julie Hicks Patrick, and Christopher J. Burant. 1997. "African American and White Mothers of Adults with Chronic Disabilities: Caregiving Burden and Satisfaction." *Family Relations* 46 (4): 335–46.

Raghavan, Chemba, Thomas S. Weisner, and Devindra Patel. 1999. "The Adaptive Project of Parenting: South Asian Families with Children with Developmental Delays." *Education and Training in Mental Retardation and Developmental Disabilities* 34 (3): 281–92.

Randall, Peter, and Jonathan Parker. 1999. *Supporting the Families of Children with Autism.* New York: John Wiley & Sons.

Rodriguez, Barbara L., and Lesley B. Olswang. 2003. "Mexican-American and Anglo-American Mothers' Beliefs and Values About Child Rearing, Education, and Language Impairment." *American Journal of Speech-Language Pathology* 12 (4): 452–62.

Rogers, Sally J. 1999. "An Examination of the Imitation Deficit in Autism." In *Imitation in Infancy,* ed. J. Nadel and G. Butterworth, 254–283. New York: Cambridge University Press.

Rogers-Dulan, Jeannette, and Jan Blacher. 1995. "African American Families, Religion, and Disability: A Conceptual Framework." *Mental Retardation* 33 (4): 226–38.

Sattler, Jerome M. 2001. *Assessment of Children: Cognitive Applications.* San Diego: Jerome M. Sattler, Publisher.

Sattler, Jerome M., and Ron Dumont. 2004. *Assessment of Children: WISC-IV and WPPSI-III Supplement.* San Diego: Jerome M. Sattler, Publisher.

Schnittker, Jason. 2003. "Misgivings of Medicine? African Americans' Skepticism of Psychiatric Medication." *Journal of Health and Social Behavior* 44 (4): 506–24.

Seligman, Milton. 1999. "Childhood Disability and the Family." In *Handbook of Psychosocial Characteristics of Exceptional Children,* ed. V. L. Schwean and D. H. Saklofske, 111–32. Dordrecht, the Netherlands: Kluwer Academic Publishers.

Shaked, Michal, and Yoram Bilu. 2006. "Grappling with Affliction: Autism in the Jewish Ultraorthodox Community in Israel." *Culture, Medicine and Psychiatry* 30 (1): 1–27.

Skinner, Debra, Donald B. Bailey Jr., Vivian Correa, and Patricia Rodriguez. 1999. "Narrating Self and Disability: Latino Mothers' Construction of Identities vis-à-vis Their Child with Special Needs." *Exceptional Children* 65 (4): 481–95.

Stevens, Gregory D., and Leiyu Shi. 2003. "Racial and Ethnic Disparities in the Primary Care Experiences of Children: A Review of the Literature." *Medical Care Research and Review* 60 (1): 3–30.

Sue, Derald Wing, and David Sue. 2008. *Counseling the Culturally Diverse: Theory and Practice (5th ed.).* Hoboken, NJ: John Wiley & Sons.

Tarakeshwar, Nalini, and Kenneth I. Pargament. 2001. "Religious Coping in Families of Children with Autism." *Focus on Autism and Other Developmental Disabilities* 16 (4): 247–60.

Terhune, Peggy S. 2005. "African-American Developmental Disability Discourses: Implications for Policy Development." *Journal of Policy and Practice in Intellectual Disabilities* 2 (1): 18–28.

Thomas, Kathleen C., Alan R. Ellis, Carolyn McLaurin, Julie Daniels, and Joseph P. Morrissey. 2007. "Access to Care for Autism-related Services." *Journal of Autism and Developmental Disorders* 37 (10): 1902–12.

Tomasello, Michael. 1992. "The Social Bases of Language Acquisition." *Social Development* 1 (1): 67–87.

Treffert, Darold A. 1970. "Epidemiology of Infantile Autism." *Archives of General Psychiatry* 22 (5): 431–38.

Tsang, Hector W. H., Phidias K. C. Tam, Fong Chan, and W. M. Cheung. 2003. "Stigmatizing Attitudes Towards Individuals with Mental Illness in Hong Kong: Implications for Their Recovery." *Journal of Community Psychology* 31 (4): 383–96.

Tsang, Sandra K. M., Daniel T. L. Shek, Lorinda L. Lam, Florence L. Y. Tang, and Penita M. P. Cheung. 2007. "Brief Report: Application of the TEACCH Program on Chinese Pre-school Children with Autism— Does Culture Make a Difference?" *Journal of Autism and Developmental Disorders* 37 (2): 390–96.

Turkheimer, Eric, Andreana Haley, Mary Waldron, Brian D'Onofrio, and Irving I. Gottesman. 2003. "Socioeconomic Status Modifies Heritability of IQ in Young Children." *Psychological Science* 14 (6): 623–28.

U.S. Census Bureau. 2008. S1701. "Poverty Status in the Past 12 Months." In *Survey: American Community Survey: Data Set: 2006–2008*

American Community Survey 3-Year Estimates. http://factfinder. census.gov/servlet/ADPTable?_bm=y&-geo_id=01000US&- qr_name=ACS_2008_3YR_G00_DP3YR5&-ds_name=&-_lang=en&- redoLog=false&-format=

Valentine, Deborah P., Suzanne McDermott, and Dinah Anderson. 1998. "Mothers of Adults with Mental Retardation: Is Race a Factor in Perceptions of Burdens and Gratifications?" *Families in Society* 79 (6): 577–84.

Wechsler, David. 2003. *The Wechsler Intelligence Scale for Children, 4th Edition*. San Antonio, TX: Psychological Corporation.

Wilder, Lynn K., Tina Taylor Dyches, Festus E. Obiakor, and Bob Algozzine. 2004. "Multicultural Perspectives on Teaching Students with Autism." *Focus on Autism and Other Developmental Disabilities* 19 (2): 105–13.

Williams, Justin H. G., Andrew Whiten, and Tulika Singh. 2004. "A Systematic Review of Action Imitation in Autistic Spectrum Disorder." *Journal of Autism and Developmental Disorders* 34 (3): 285–99.

Wing, Lorna. 1980. "Childhood Autism and Social Class: A Question of Selection?" *British Journal of Psychiatry* 137:410–17.

Yeh, May, Richard L. Hough, Kristen McCabe, Anna Lau, and Ann Garland. 2004. "Parental Beliefs about the Causes of Child Problems: Exploring Racial/Ethnic Patterns." *Journal of the American Academy of Child and Adolescent Psychiatry* 43 (5): 605.

4

Chronology

This chapter provides a timeline of events that have shaped our understanding and awareness of autism. Although individuals lived with what was later termed *autism* prior to the initial usage of the term, the diagnosis itself was not established until the mid-20th century. Therefore, the field of autism is relatively young compared to other mental health disorders and dates back only to the early 1900s. This chapter describes important scientific findings in autism as well as different evolutions of diagnostic criteria, events that influenced the public's awareness of the disorder, popularities of various treatments, and important events involved in examining the potential causes of autism.

1910	The Swiss psychiatrist Eugen Bleuler first uses the word *autism* to describe individuals with schizophrenia who have lost contact with reality. Dr. Bleuler describes an "autistic withdrawal of the patient to his fantasies." He adapts the word autism from the Greek word *autos*, which means "self."
1912	Dr. Bleuler publishes "Das Autistische Denken" in a journal of psychiatry and presents his thoughts on how a person with autism (as he defined autism) experiences the world.
1938	Dr. Hans Asperger, a professor of pediatrics at the University Children's Hospital in Vienna, Austria, presents a lecture on child psychology.

1938 (*cont.*)	In the lecture, he adapts Bleuler's term, *autism*, and uses the phrase "autistic psychopathy" to describe children showing social withdrawal and overly intense preoccupations.
1943	Dr. Leo Kanner, a child psychiatrist, from Johns Hopkins University, describes a childhood disorder involving social and language impairments and the presence of restricted or repetitive behaviors. He reports that the children have a similar loss of contact with reality as described by Bleuler, but do not also have schizophrenia. He describes an "extreme autistic aloneness" and coins the term "early infantile autism."
1944	Dr. Hans Asperger reports on four children with a pattern of behaviors he terms "autistic psychopathy." The behaviors included reduced empathy, difficulties with forming friendships, impairments in the ability to maintain reciprocal conversations, all encompassing interests, and clumsiness.
1950s	Psychoanalytic theories dominate the field of psychology and behavioral disorders with no identifiable medical cause, such as behavior change following a head injury, are attributed to early developmental relationships, particularly with parental figures. In the case of autism, cold, aloof parenting is attributed to the cause of the disorder.
1952	The first edition of the *Diagnostic and Statistical Manual of Mental Disorders* (*DSM*) is published. The text provides a glossary of descriptions of diagnostic categories of mental disorders. Although autism is not listed as a diagnosis, the diagnostic term *schizophrenic reaction, childhood type* is listed and is used to capture children that present with behaviors that resemble what would now be called autism.
1962	LSD is used as a treatment for "autistic schizophrenic children" and the results are reported in *Biological Psychiatry*. The authors of the study

conclude that the patients showed few side effects, appeared to be happier and "high," were more interactive with others, and showed less repetitive behavior.

The Autistic Children's Aid Society of North London (later deemed the National Autistic Society) is founded by parents of children with autism in England, including Dr. Lorna Wing, a psychiatrist who would become a prominent figure in the autism world. The initial goals are to establish a center to care for affected children, with a more general goal of creating a sound entity to represent the interests of children with autism. In the years after its inception, the organization has expanded to include chapters throughout the United Kingdom.

1964   Dr. Bernard Rimland, an experimental psychologist and parent of a child with autism, publishes *Infantile Autism*. In the book, Dr. Rimland argues that there is no evidence to support the conclusion that autism's cause is rooted in parenting. In the text, Dr. Rimland reviews what is known about autism and promotes the notion that the disorder is brain based, citing physiological evidence and implicating genetics.

1965   Dr. Bernard Rimland and Dr. Ruth Sullivan join forces with other parents of children with autism to found the National Society for Autistic Children (later named Autism Society of America) in the United States. The core founders of the nonprofit foundation gather in response to the flood of support letters following the publication of *Infantile Autism* and Dr. Rimland's refutation that poor parenting causes autism. The mission of the organization is to improve the lives of all individuals with autism.

Life magazine publishes a story about the treatment employed by Ivar Lovaas, professor of psychology at the University of California at Los Angeles. The article titled, "Screams, Slaps

1965 (*cont.*)	& Love: A Surprising, Shocking Treatment Helps Far-gone Mental Cripples," provides a description of the treatment, based on the principles of Applied Behavioral Analysis. The treatment is the first to be scientifically studied and empirically validated to be effective in ameliorating symptoms.
1967	Dr. Bernard Rimland founds the Autism Research Institute (ARI) in San Diego, California, with the mission to improve diagnosis, treatment, and prevention of autism through scientific research. Dr. Rimland remains involved in the organization until his death in 2006. The organization holds conferences called "Defeat Autism Now!" and is known for its focus on biomedical treatments of autism.
	Dr. Bruno Bettelheim, a professor of psychology at the University of Chicago and director of the Sonia Shankman Orthogenic School for treating children with developmental disabilities, publishes his book, *The Empty Fortress: Infantile Autism and the Birth of the Self*. In accordance with the psychodynamic context of that time period, he proposes that autism is caused by "rejecting parents." The book contains Dr. Bettelheim's most cited statement, "Throughout this book I state my belief that the precipitating factor in infantile autism is the parent's wish that his child should not exist."
1968	The second edition of the *Diagnostic and Statistical Manual of Mental Disorders* is published. Under the diagnostic category *schizophrenia, childhood type*, autism is included as a descriptor.
1971	Professor of psychology, Dr. Eric Schopler, at the University of North Carolina, proposes that instead of treating parents of children with autism, therapists should involve parents as part of treatment for the child. He publishes the manuscript: "Parents as Cotherapists in the Treatment of Psychotic Children."

The *Journal of Autism and Childhood Schizophenia* (later renamed *Journal of Autism and Developmental Disorders*) is founded with Leo Kanner as the editor in chief. The first issue includes articles by Drs. Leo Kanner, Michael Rutter, and Eric Schopler.

1972   Dr. Eric Schopler founds Division TEACCH (Treatment and Education of Autistic and related Communication-handicapped Children), a program that focuses on providing a structured teaching environment and including parents as cotherapists to aid in the treatment and education of children with autism. The program was originally developed through a research grant and parents involved in the study, along with Dr. Schopler, successfully petition the state legislature for permanent funding.

1977   Dr. Susan Folstein and Sir Michael Rutter, both prominent child psychiatrists, publish findings from a twin study of autism conducted in the United Kingdom. By comparing the concordance rates for autism in identical and fraternal twins, they demonstrate that autism is a genetic disorder, ending the myth that autism is caused by "cold, aloof, refrigerator" mothers.

1979   Lorna Wing, a psychiatrist and parent of a daughter with autism, collaborates with Judith Gould, a clinical psychologist, to publish their findings on the prevalence of autism and their hypothesis that the pattern of behaviors previously termed *infantile autism* is really a spectrum of disorders. The term *autism spectrum* is born.

1980   Autism is considered a rare childhood disorder. The prevalence of autism is estimated at 4 in 10,000 children.

The third edition of the *DSM* is published. For the first time autism is identified as a disorder of its own right, separate from childhood schizophrenia. The term *infantile autism* is used to describe

1980 (*cont.*)	"a pervasive lack of responsiveness to other people," deficits in language development, peculiar speech patterns, bizarre responses to various aspects of the environment, and the absence of delusions or hallucinations as seen in schizophrenia.
1981	Dr. Lorna Wing popularizes Dr. Hans Asperger's research and writings and champions the idea that Asperger's Disorder, termed *Asperger's Syndrome* in the publication, is a separate and distinct subtype of pervasive developmental disorder from Autistic Disorder. Much debate regarding the existence of distinct subtypes and whether or not Asperger's Disorder and Autistic Disorder are separate disorders ensues in the scientific community. The debate continues today.
	Dr. O. Ivar Lovaas publishes a book geared toward parents called *Teaching Developmentally Disabled Children: The Me Book*. The book is a training manual that provides detailed explanations and examples of how to apply the principles of behavior therapy. It is designed for use with children with a variety of challenges, including autism, mental retardation, and brain damage.
1985	Working under the mentorship of Dr. Uta Frith, doctoral student Simon Baron-Cohen conducts studies examining deficits in "theory of mind" in children with autism. *Theory of mind* is a term adapted from work with chimpanzee cognition and refers to the cognitive ability to understand that other people have beliefs, intentions, and wishes that are different from one's own intentions and beliefs. The initial tasks used to assess theory of mind were easy to administer and have spawned a vast field of research in autism as well as in typical development.
1987	The revision of the third edition of the *Diagnostic and Statistical Manual of Mental Disorders* (*DSM-III-R*) is published. In this edition, the term

infantile autism is replaced by Autistic Disorder, and additional specific criteria are included regarding the disorder. Criteria for Pervasive Developmental Disorder are specified to indicate that this category refers to children with significant social and language impairments but who do not meet criteria for another disorder.

Dr. Ivar Lovaas, at the University of California, Los Angeles publishes the results of a study demonstrating the effectiveness of applying behavioral principles (termed *Applied Behavior Analysis*, or ABA) to treatment for children with autism. The intervention entails approximately 40 hours per week of repeated trials (called discrete trial training) in which the child with autism is reinforced through rewards for correct performance. He reports finding significant improvements in intelligence scores for children and highlights that many of the children receiving intervention in the study are placed in regular education classrooms.

1988   Dustin Hoffman wins an Oscar for his portrayal of Raymond Babbit in the movie *Rainman*. Babbit is a man with autism who shows marked impairments in social interactions, savant mathematical skills, ritualized behaviors, and a crippling insistence on sameness. For the first time, the word *autism* becomes popularized and awareness of the disorder increases among the general public.

1989   Dr. Douglas Biklen, a psychologist at Syracuse University, returns from a trip to Melbourne Australia where he observed an assisted technology called Facilitated Communication (FC) developed by a teacher, Rosemary Crossley, as a result of her work with individuals with cerebral palsy in the 1970s. Dr. Biklen popularizes FC in the United States as a way to help individuals with autism communicate via a keyboard with a facilitator touching the individual's hands while he/she typed. Viewed as a miracle tool by

1989 (*cont.*)	parents of nonverbal children with autism, FC achieves rapid, widespread use despite no evidence of its effectiveness.
	Dr. Catherine Lord, a professor of psychology and autism expert, and colleagues publish a standardized observation of communication and social behaviors called the *Autism Diagnostic Observation Schedule*. Soon after its publication, it is widely used as a diagnostic tool in both clinical and research in autism and is important because it allows for a standardized comparison of children across study samples.
	Drs. Michael Rutter, Ann LeCouteur, and Catherine Lord publish an interview for parents of children with autism (or suspected autism), called the Autism Diagnostic Interview (ADI). Primarily used in research settings due to its length, it helps to standardize information obtained about current and past behaviors in children with autism. It was later revised in 1994 to reflect new diagnostic criteria for autism spectrum disorders.
1993	Through FC, Betsy Wheaton, a child with autism, reports that her parents, grandparents and brother have sexually abused her. This allegation prompts studies of the FC as a legitimate means of communicating to be conducted. Subsequent studies find time and time again that it is the facilitator who is doing the communicating, not the children and FC is found to be an invalid means of allowing children to communicate.
1994	Julie Osterling, a graduate student at the University of Washington, and her mentor, professor of psychology Dr. Geraldine Dawson, publish the findings of home videotapes of first year birthday parties of children later diagnosed with autism and children with typical development. The authors show that children with autism can be differentiated from typically developing children at one year of age due to reduced eye con-

tact, response to name and pointing and showing behaviors. This finding indicates that children with autism can be identified several years before concerns are assessed and they are diagnosed in the community.

The fourth edition of the *DSM* is published. Pervasive Developmental Disorders (PDD) is listed as an umbrella term that encompasses five distinct disorders: Autistic Disorder, Asperger's Disorder, Rett's Syndrome, Childhood Disintegrative Disorder, and Pervasive Developmental Disorders—Not Otherwise Specified. In this edition of the *DSM*, Asperger's Disorder becomes a distinct disorder.

Committees updating the Pervasive Developmental Disorders section of the *DSM* collaborate with committees developing the ninth edition of the *International Classification of Diseases*, which allows for the establishment of identical diagnostic criteria for both manuals. This creates a worldwide standard for PDDs allowing research and clinical information to be translated across continents.

Frustrated by the slow pace of scientific progress regarding ASDs and the limited research funds dedicated to autism research by the National Institutes of Health, Karen and Eric London, parents of a child with autism, found National Alliance for Autism Research (NAAR) to become first nonprofit devoted to furthering autism research. Through funds garnered by parent donations, the organization supports research into the causes and treatments of autism. NAAR goes on to establish the Autism Tissue Program to collect postmortem brains of individuals with autism to study the underlying anatomical and cellular features of autism.

1995   Jonathan Shestack and Portia Iversen, parents of a child with autism, found Cure Autism Now (CAN), a parent-based funding organization

1995 (*cont.*)   dedicated to autism research. Both CAN and NAAR increase public awareness of autism and provide funds for increasing awareness and advancing research.

A team of researchers in the United Kingdom led by Anthony Bailey report their findings from an expansion of the 1977 Folstein and Rutter seminal twin study. With a true population-based sample ascertained by contacting every school, clinic, and twin register in the country and all cases of autism verified with standardized parent report and child observation, this well-conducted study further clarifies the role of genetics in autism and replicates the original findings of an increased concordance rate for identical twins than fraternal twins. Furthermore, these newer findings suggest an even higher concordance rate for identical twins than the original 1977 paper.

1997   The National Institutes of Child Health and Development establish the Collaborative Programs for Excellence in Autism (CPEA) and provide $105 million in research funding over 10 years to nine network sites, including Boston University, the University of California at Davis, the University of California at Los Angeles, the University of Washington, the University of Rochester Medical Center, the University of Utah, the University of Michigan, the University of Pittsburg, and Yale University. Each center conducts its own projects in autism focusing on genetics, neuroscience, early identification, early development, and treatment. A standardization of a portion of measures allows for collaboration and data sharing, thereby increasing the number of participants in the study nationwide.

Soon after establishing CAN, Portia Iversen and Jonathan Shestack cofound the Autism Genetics Resource Exchange (AGRE), the world's largest gene bank open to the scientific community to help search for genetic influences in autism.

Prominent genetics researchers are recruited to work on AGRE.

1998   First genome-wide linkage analysis of autism is published in a well-known genetics journal by a global scientific group, the International Molecular Genetic Study of Autism Consortium, suggesting a chromosomal hotspot for autism on chromosome 7. Other chromosomal areas, including chromosome 16, are also found to be significant. The study examined 99 families containing family members affected with autism and it represents an important step toward identifying autism predisposition genes.

After his son is diagnosed with autism, Doug Flutie, former NFL quarterback, founds the Doug Flutie Jr. Foundation for Autism. Its goal is to provide funding directly to families to help with treatment costs and also provides small grants to treatment research.

Dr. Andrew Wakefield publishes findings in a leading general medical journal (*The Lancet*) reporting cases of 12 children with developmental disabilities who have traces of measles mRNA in the gut. This finding fuels fire to the idea that autism is caused by immunizations, particularly the MMR vaccine, and is considered by those in support of the autism-vaccine connection to represent significant scientific support for their claim. After the publication of this study, rates of inoculation in England drop from 92 percent to below 80 percent.

First Signs Inc. is founded by a parent of a child with autism and is a national nonprofit organization whose mission is to promote the best outcome for children through early identification of challenges. The organization has worked diligently to improve screening processes for young children with the goal to lower the age at which children are diagnosed with autism. Among other resources, their Web site contains a video glossary of early warning signs of autism.

1999	The hormone Secretin is reported on a population television show *Dateline* to have miraculously cured one child's autism. Secretin is a peptide hormone that is used during a medical procedure called an endoscopy to test pancreatic functioning and is not FDA-approved for any use other than as a diagnostic aid in endoscopies. Although subsequent studies indicate no effectiveness of Secretin, many parents seek out doctors who will prescribe Secretin to treat their child's autism and prices for Secretin soar due to the high demand.
Late 1990s	Conclusions from Dr. Wakefield's paper are subsequently retracted by 10 of the 13 authors on the paper. *The Lancet* later retracts the manuscript when it is revealed that Dr. Wakefield is being retained by families and attorneys in lawsuits against a vaccine company.
2000s	Parents and advocacy groups across the country lobby state congresses to mandate insurance companies to cover the cost of such autism treatments as ABA, which can be more than $70,000–$90,000 for the recommended 25 hours/week of individual therapy. Some states pass the laws, including Arizona, Pennsylvania, and South Carolina, but include a cap of $36,000–50,000 per year for insurance coverage of treatments. Insurance companies claim that autism treatments are educational in nature, not medical, and lack strong evidence of effectiveness.
	Jenny McCarthy, among many other parents of children with autism, continues to call for a closer examination of a causal relationship between vaccines and autism, despite continued opposing reports from the Institute of Medicine. Recommendations include a major overhaul in the national immunization schedule and in the compounds used in vaccines.
2000	Talking About Curing Autism (TACA) is founded and promotes biomedical treatments for chil-

dren with autism. Jenny McCarthy partners with this organization after her son is diagnosed with autism.

Portia Iversen establishes the International Meeting for Autism Research (IMFAR) to create a forum to present research findings specific to autism. The first IMFAR conference is held in San Diego, California, in 2001. IMFAR continues to be held annually in different cities across the world and is the most attended and popular scientific conference specific to autism.

President Bill Clinton signs the Children's Health Act and founds an autism research coordinating committee. Among other goals, the Children's Health Act directs federal agencies to study diseases that are increasingly prevalent in the United States, including autism.

The Children's Health Act mandates that the National Institutes for Mental Health dedicate $65 million to establishing the Studies to Advance Autism Research and Treatment (STAART network) and eight STAART centers are established across the United States: Boston University; Kennedy Krieger Institute; Mt. Sinai Medical School; University of California, Los Angeles; University of North Carolina, Chapel Hill; University of Rochester; University of Washington; and Yale University. Each center supports three or more research projects, with at least one study focused on treatment, and engage in multisite clinical trials and collaborations. Most of the studies conducted at the centers evaluate and treat patients, as well as enroll them into clinical trials.

2001   U.S. Rep, Christopher Smith (R-NJ) and Rep. Mike Doyle (D-PA) found the Congressional Autism Caucus, also known as the Congressional Coalition for Autism Research & Education (C.A.R.E.). The bipartisan caucus goes on to

2001 (*cont.*) include more than 160 members of Congress and is the first organization in Congress to focus its efforts on autism spectrum disorders.

The Institute of Medicine publishes the first of eight Immunization Safety Reviews, three of which pertain directly to autism. In this first report, available published and unpublished scientific evidence are reviewed and the committee concludes that there is no causal link between immunizations and autism at a general population level. The report also concludes that Dr. Wakefield's paper is "uninformative with respect to causality between MMR and ASD" due to the small number of children included in the study, multiple diagnoses of the sample, selection bias, and the lack of detail about diagnoses of the children in the study.

In the second report of the Immunization Safety Review, the Institute of Medicine concludes that the relationship between thimerosal-containing vaccines and the onset of neurodevelopmental disorders such as autism and ADHD is not established and research support is indirect and incomplete. Nevertheless, thimerosal is recommended to be removed from the vaccinations DTaP, Hib, and hepatitis B vaccines in the United States. These vaccinations remain thimerosal-free today.

2002 Further work at the University of Washington utilizing a home videotape study demonstrates that children with autism can be differentiated from children with mental retardation as early as 12 months of age. Social behaviors that distinguish infants with developmental delay versus autism included orienting to name, looking at people, and frequency of directed vocalizations. People watching the videotapes use these three factors alone to correctly classify 87 percent of 12-month-old infants in the study as either going on to be diagnosed with autism or developmental delay.

2003   Jim and Marilyn Simons from the Simons Foundation decide to take on a new initiative in their organization to fund autism research. A new direction from their focus on basic science and mathematics research, they call prominent autism researchers together to meet about up-and-coming topics and next steps in the field. The Simons Foundation goes on to dedicate more than $100 million to autism research in subsequent years.

2004   This eighth and final Immunization Safety Review report determines that the "body of epidemiological evidence favors rejection of a causal relationship between the MMR vaccine and autism. The committee also concludes that the body of epidemiological evidence favors rejection of a causal relationship between thimerosal-containing vaccines and autism." Potential biological mechanisms for vaccine-induced autism are determined to be plausible in theory, but not supported by the numerous scientific studies conducted to date.

2005   The nonprofit foundation Autism Speaks is founded by Suzanne and Bob Wright (former CEO of the television network NBC) who are grandparents of a child with autism. Autism Speaks has raised $200 million to date and is known for lobbying congress and private citizens to allocate research money and national attention to autism. Now the nation's leading nonprofit organization devoted to autism, Autism Speaks plays a key role in the successful passage of the Combating Autism Act and is a primary player in placing autism on the United Nations global health agenda.

Average age of diagnosis for autism drops nationally to approximately 3 years of age, with some research institutions, including some STAART centers, beginning to diagnosis children at 18 months of age. Mandell and colleagues report in the medical journal *Pediatrics* that the

2005 (*cont.*)   average age of diagnosis is 3.1 years for children with Autistic Disorder, 3.9 years for PDD-NOS, and 7.2 years for Asperger's Disorder (Mandell et al. 2005. "Factors Associated with Age of Diagnosis among Children with Autism Spectrum Disorders." *Pediatrics* 116 (6): 148086).

2006   National Alliance for Autism Research (NAAR) merges with Autism Speaks. Karen and Eric London (NAAR's cofounders) remain actively involved in the organization's growth and development.

The Combating Autism Act is signed into law by President George W. Bush. This legislation authorizes nearly one billion dollars in government expenditures, over a five-year period, to be put toward screening, education, early intervention, prompt referrals for treatment and services, and research in the autism spectrum disorders. This amount is approximately double the existing budget for these areas of focus and allows for additional Autism Centers of Excellence to be funded.

2007   The U.S. Senate designates April as National Autism Awareness Month.

Numerous publications of epidemiological studies, both with cohort and ecological designs, as well as scientifically designed experiments, all fail to find evidence for causative link between immunizations and autism. As immunization rates fall and thimerosal or ethylmercury (preservatives used in vaccines) are removed from vaccines, autism rates continue to rise.

Autism Speaks merges with Cure Autism Now to form the largest nonprofit autism advocacy group in the nation. Autism Speaks' global influence continues to rise.

Prevalence of autism spectrum disorders is estimated to be 1 in 150 children in the United States by the Centers for Disease Control and Prevention, which is a very substantial increase from previous prevalence rates reported in autism. Scientists suggest that the loosening of diagnostic criteria, changes in ascertainment and study design, earlier detection, and increased awareness lead to much of the increases in prevalence rates, but that there does appear to be some secular increase in the rate of autism. ASDs are now considered one of the most common developmental disabilities in children.

The National Institutes for Health establishes a network of research institutions called the Autism Centers of Excellence (ACE) to serve as a consolidation of the CPEA and STAART networks. The ACE program encompasses research centers and research networks. ACE Center award recipients are University of Illinois at Chicago; University of California, San Diego; University of Washington; University of Pittsburgh; and University of California, Los Angeles; and ACE network award recipients are University of North Carolina at Chapel Hill and University of California Davis.

Jenny McCarthy publishes her book *Louder Than Words: A Mother's Journey in Healing Autism* and begins appearing on such national television shows as *Oprah*, relaying the story of her son's recovery from autism through biomedical treatments such as the gluten- and casein-free diet. She and fellow actor Jim Carrey, take a strong stand in favor of the link between autism and vaccines.

Jonathan Sebat and Michael Wigler, along with many other authors, publish a groundbreaking genetics article in one of the most prestigious scientific journals in the world: *Science*. Sebat and colleagues report that a specific type of genetic mutation called copy number variants (CNVs) occur significantly more often in children with autism who do not have a family history of the disorder (simplex families, sporadic autism) as

2007 (*cont.*)   compared to children without autism *and* compared to children with autism from families containing more than one child with autism (multiplex families, familial autism). Sebat's article sparks a new line of genetic research in the field of autism examining simplex families and is considered groundbreaking because it suggests that familial and sporadic autism may develop from different genetic mechanisms.

Based on findings from the study by Sebat et al. (2007), the Simons Simplex Collection Project (SSC) begins. The SSC is a multisite genetics study funded by the Simons Foundation that includes 11 sites in the United States and Canada. Two additional sites are added in the next year with the goal of collecting 3,000 simplex families to further explore genetic mechanisms of sporadic autism.

2008   One additional ACE program Center is awarded to Yale University. Additional ACE program network award recipients are Wayne State University; University of California, Los Angeles; and Drexel University.

2009   Dr. Wakefield and two coauthors on his paper (Professor John Walker-Smith and Professor Simon Murch) are under investigation for falsifying data in their 1998 paper that sparked the controversial belief that the MMR vaccine causes autism. A careful examination of the medical records of the patients included in Dr. Wakefield's study suggest that the symptoms described in the children's medical records do not correspond with the those reported in Dr. Wakefield's research article and that some of the symptoms reported as having an onset *after* the MMR vaccine were actually documented in the children's medical records *before* the immunization was given. If the results of this investigation are true, it rules out the possibility that the vaccines could have caused the symptoms since they were present before the immunization was given.

Alison Singer resigns as executive vice president of Autism Speaks due to her disagreement with the organization's continued pursuit of research into the link between autism and vaccines despite repeated studies demonstrating no relationship. She then founds her own nonprofit called the Autism Science Foundation whose mission is to support research in autism, particularly genetic influences. Karen London, cofounder of NAAR, also joins the organization.

Months after Alison Singer leaves Autism Speaks, Dr. Eric London, cofounder of the autism research foundation NAAR, resigns from his role on the Autism Speaks Scientific Affairs Committee Speaks. In his resignation letter, he states "the pivotal issue compelling my decision is the position which Autism Speaks is taking concerning vaccinations. The arguments which Dr. Dawson [Chief Scientific Officer of Autism Speaks] and others assert—that the parents need even further assurances and there might be rare cases of 'biologically plausible' vaccine involvement—are misleading and disingenuous."

5

Biographical Sketches

This chapter will provide brief biographies of notable individuals whose work and/or lives are relevant to the field of autism. Individuals discussed are autism researchers, founders of autism nonprofit organizations, and influential figures in increasing autism awareness to the general public. Their various contributions to the autism community will be discussed in detail and noteworthy background information about their training and introduction into autism will be included, if pertinent. Wherever possible, birth years and year of death will be stated. This list is not exhaustive and we have attempted to sample individuals from a variety of disciplines to provide as much breadth as possible.

Hans Asperger (1906–1980)

Hans Asperger was born on a farm in Austria and the elder of two sons. He showed a talent for language and loved to memorize and recite poetry. His favorite poet was Franz Grillparzer, the Austrian national poet. He did not make friends easily in his early years, but did so during the 1920s when he became involved in the youth movement in Austria. He studied medicine in Vienna and in 1931 graduated with a medical doctorate. During World War II, he served as a medical officer in Croatia. After the war he took the position of chair of pediatrics at the University Children's Hospital in Vienna. In 1944 he described four children with "autistic psychopathy." He used the term to describe the pattern of behaviors that included reduced empathy, difficulties with forming friendships and maintaining reciprocal conversations, all encompassing interests, and clumsiness. He highlighted their strengths in intellectual ability and curiosity and likened the children to "little professors." Dr. Asperger is known for highlighting the strengths of his patients and this is true in his descriptions of the children. It has been suggested that his focusing on the positive aspects of the behaviors is because, he, himself had Asperger's Disorder. Dr. Asperger was tirelessly devoted to the field and although there was little mention of Asperger's Disorder prior to the 1994 inclusion of the disorder in the *Diagnostic and Statistical Manual*, the size of his contribution to the field is now clear.

Tony Attwood (b. 1952)

Tony Attwood, PhD, is a British psychologist who has authored several bestselling books on ASD, particularly on Asperger's Disorder. Two of his books are *Asperger's Syndrome: A Guide for Parents and Professionals* and *The Complete Guide to Asperger's Syndrome*. Dr. Attwood has an honors degree in psychology from the University of Hull, a master's degree in clinical psychology from the University of Surrey, and a doctorate from the University of London, working under Dr. Uta Frith. He currently resides in Queensland, Australia, and is an adjunct associate professor at Griffith University in Queensland. Clinical work continues to be important to Dr. Attwood, and he has a diagnostic and treatment clinic for children and adults with autism in Brisbane, Australia. His research has been largely focused on treatment, and he has recently published articles reporting positive effects of cognitive behavioral therapy for managing associated symptoms (anxiety and anger) of Asperger's Disorder.

Dr. Attwood first became interested in autism in 1971 while working as a volunteer at a school for special needs. After meeting two young children with autism, he became dedicated to understanding their unusual behavior and helping children and adults with autism in whatever way he could. Since then, Dr. Attwood's career has been largely focused on helping individuals with Asperger's Disorder throughout the lifespan, including adulthood and elderly populations.

Simon Baron-Cohen (b. 1958)

Professor Baron-Cohen made a significant contribution to the understanding of autism and the field of developmental psychology when he authored the first publication indicating deficits and delays in "theory of mind" in individuals with autism. The paper was the result of his research conducted during his graduate work. *Theory of mind* is a term adapted from the study of cognitive processes in chimpanzees and refers to the cognitive ability to understand that others have beliefs, intentions, and wishes that are different from one's own intentions and beliefs. His initial publication on "theory of mind" spawned a vast field of research in autism as well as in typical development. Following his pioneering work into the theory of mind, Dr. Baron-Cohen developed a theory to explain the gender differences observed in autism. He proposed that autism is a form of the extreme male brain. This theory has been met with both support and skepticism by the scientific community. Dr. Baron-Cohen holds a PhD in psychology from University College in London, a master's degree in clinical psychology from the Institute of Psychiatry, as well as a master's degree in human sciences. He is currently a professor of developmental psychopathology at the University of Cambridge and director of the Autism Research Center. His cousin is the comedic actor Sacha Baron-Cohen, known for his roles in *Da Ali G* show and the movie *Borat.*

Margaret Bauman (dates unknown)

Margaret Bauman, MD, pioneered an understanding of the biological basis of autism with her work identifying anatomical abnormalities in brain structures in individuals of autism. In addition to her research in the biology of autism, she is a clinician who has led the movement toward a multidisciplinary approach to the treatment of autism. She founded LADDERS (Learning and Developmental Disabilities and Rehabilitation Services) in 1981 to provide comprehensive diagnostic and treatment services that focus on the integration of disciplines ranging from neurology, gastroenterology, social work, physical therapy, occupational therapy, psychiatry, psychology, speech therapy, nursing, and genetics to help individuals with autism and developmental disabilities achieve their full potential. The Autism Treatment Network, funded by Autism Speaks, is in part based on her clinic and treatment approach at LADDERS, located at Massachusetts General Hospital, and she has served as the medical director the network.

In addition to directing LADDERS, Dr. Bauman is an associate professor of neurology at Harvard University Medical School and an adjunct associate professor of anatomy and neurobiology at Boston University School of Medicine. In 1990 she started and organized the Autism Research Fund (TARF) to underscore the important role that research with brains of individuals with autism can play in identifying the pathophysiology of the disorder. Since that time a large number of individuals with autism have donated their brains for autopsy and research to allow for this type of research.

Bruno Bettelheim (1903–1990)

Bruno Bettelheim was best known for his writings regarding autism and his belief that autism was caused by cold, aloof "refrigerator" mothering. He was born in Austria and began his education at the University of Vienna. With the death of his father he withdrew from his studies to manage his family's sawmill although he later returned to Vienna to finish his education. Dr. Bettelheim was Jewish and shortly after completing his dissertation in art history he was sent to a concentration camp in 1938. He regained his freedom in 1939 with a number of other prisoners following an amnesty that was granted. He emigrated to New York to reunite with his wife, who had emigrated earlier, but she had already become involved with another man. As a result he moved to Chicago and quickly took a position in psychology. He taught at Chicago University from 1944 until his retirement in 1973. While in Chicago he also directed the Sonia Shankman Orthogenic School and based much of his writings on his experiences treating children with emotional disturbances. He published a number of books during his tenure at the University of Chicago, most notably, *The Empty Fortress: Infantile Autism and the Birth of the Self,* which fostered the refrigerator mother theory. Biographies published after his suicide in 1990 indicate that many of his reported accomplishments were fabricated, including his multiple degrees, his academic awards, his positive reviews by Freud, training experiences, the care and improvement of the children he worked with at the Orthogenic School, and even his reported involvement with the anti-Nazi underground.

Eugene Bleuler (1857–1939)

Eugene Bleuler was born in Switzerland and studied medicine in Zurich, Paris, London, and Munich. In the late 1880s and early 1890s he served as director of the psychiatric clinic at the hospital Rheinau and made significant improvements in patient care. In 1898 he became director of the Burgholzli, the psychiatric hospital at the University of Zurich. One of his interns was Carl Jung, the psychiatrist who started the Jungian branch of psychology. Dr. Bleuler is credited with renaming dementia praecox as schizophrenia. Basing on the Greek word *schizein*, which means "split," and *phren*, which means "mind," Dr. Bleuler suggested this was a better descriptor for the disorder. He presented in a speech at the German Psychiatric Association in Berlin that the disorder was not a form of dementia and most often developed in early adulthood and was therefore not an early developing disorder (*praecox* meaning "early"). In a 1910 paper on schizophrenia, Dr. Bleuler discussed the "autistic withdrawal of the patient to his fantasies, again which any influence from outside sources becomes and intolerable disturbance." He adapted the word autism from the Greek word *autos*, meaning "self." It was the first time that the word *autism* was used in print to refer to mental illness. Two years later, in 1912, Dr. Bleuler published an article, "Das Autistische Denken," in a journal of psychiatry, and in it he muses on the world of an autistic person. This 1912 text focuses on Dr. Bleuler's concept of autism and is not used in the same sense that it is currently.

Tony Charman (dates unknown)

Tony Charman, PhD, is a clinical psychologist based at the Institute of Health in London where he is a professor of Autism Education and Neurodevelopmental Disorders. His research has focused on the early social cognitive development in children with autism spectrum disorders, including examinations of imitation abilities in young children with autism and children who experienced a regression in language early in life. Recent work from Dr. Charman's research group involves studying varying cognitive abilities of children with autism. Dr. Charman is also a well-known clinician and his research has remained firmly grounded in his clinical work at the Great Ormond Street Hospital for Children in the United Kingdom. His clinical research interests have included the development of screening tools to aid in the early identification of autism spectrum disorders, epidemiological studies, intervention studies, and the prospective study of infants who are at risk for developing autism. Dr. Charman has also published a number of research articles refuting the purported link between the measles vaccination and autism. Dr. Charman was the editor-in-chief of the *Journal of Child Psychology and Psychiatry* between 2007 and 2009 and has been associate editor and contributor to a number of other scientific journals, including *Autism Research* and *Journal of Autism and Developmental Disorders*.

Eric Courchesne (dates unknown)

Eric Courchesne, PhD, is a neuroscientist whose work has focused on studying the brain functioning and neuroanatomy of individuals with autism. Dr. Courchesne is currently a Professor of Neuroscience at the University of California San Diego (UCSD) Medical School and director of the UCSD Autism Center of Excellence (ACE) awarded by the National Institute of Mental Health. He has published over 140 scientific articles in his academic career. Among many other research findings on specific brain regions implicated in autism, Dr. Courchesne was the first to document abnormally large brains in young children with autism (2–3 years of age) compared to both typically developing children and those with developmental delays without autism. The overgrowth is most notable in neural systems involved in cognitive, language, emotional and social functions that are known to be impaired in autism.

Dr. Courchesne's work has also extended down to infancy and his laboratory carefully documented abnormal head circumference growth trajectories in infants who go on to be diagnosed with autism. Head circumference is considered to be a good estimate of overall brain size and volume in children. Dr. Courchesne obtained this information by examining medical records and head circumference measurements at well-baby visits with pediatricians. He found that newborns who go on to be diagnosed with autism, on average, have normal to slightly below normal sized heads in the first one to two months of life. This period is followed by a rapid growth in head circumference during the first year of life, which levels off and approaches a normal growth trajectory in the second year of life. These findings were significant in the field of autism because they documented neurological abnormalities present in individuals with autism before a diagnosis was made and generally before behavioral differences were noted. Overall, it lends support to the conceptualization of autism as a developmental disorder with a divergence from typical development detectable in infancy.

Geraldine Dawson (b. 1951)

Geraldine Dawson, PhD, is a well-known autism researcher who retired in 2008 from a long career in academia and is now working as Chief Science Officer at the autism advocacy organization *Autism Speaks*. Dr. Dawson is a clinical psychologist and completed her undergraduate and graduate work at the University of Washington and received her doctorate degree in 1979. She is the founding director of the University of Washington Autism Center and Professor Emeritus of Psychology at the University of Washington. Dr. Dawson was the director of the University of Washington Center of Excellence in Autism Research as well as the director of the Collaborative Program of Excellence in Autism from the mid-1990s through 2008.

Dr. Dawson has conducted research in many areas within the field of autism, including autism diagnosis, brain functioning, genetics, early identification of autism and, more recently, intervention and prevention. She has authored five books on autism and has published more than 150 research articles in her academic career. Important research findings from Dr. Dawson include discoveries of abnormal face processing in the brains of individuals with autism and further research into the social brain circuitry involved in autism. Her laboratory also conducted home videotape studies validating early indicators of autism in infancy and providing substantial support for the authenticity of autistic regression. Dr. Dawson has contributed greatly to the understanding of the genetic underpinnings of autism and to the features of the broader autism phenotype in family members of children with autism. In addition to scientific contributions, Dr. Dawson testified before the U.S. Senate on behalf of individuals with autism and was a leading member of the Washington State Autism Task Force.

Susan Folstein (b. 1944)

Dr. Susan Folstein has been an active researcher in the field of psychiatry since the 1970s. She received her MD at Cornell Medical College in 1970. Following her medical education at Cornell, internship in pediatrics at Bronx Municipal Hospital and residency in child psychiatry at New York Hospital, Dr. Folstein sought out further training with Sir Michael Rutter at Maudsley Hospital in London. As a fellow under the guidance of Professor Rutter, Dr. Folstein conducted a twin study of autism and definitively demonstrated that autism is a genetic disorder. Her findings, published in 1977, struck a significant blow to the refrigerator mother theory of autism. Following her return from the United Kingdom, Dr. Folstein took a position as professor of psychiatry at Johns Hopkins University. There she continued her work in the field of psychiatric genetics including work on Huntington's Disease as well as autism. In collaboration with her husband, Dr. Marshall Folstein, Dr. Susan Folstein developed the mini mental status exam, an easy to administer tool for physicians to assess the mental status of psychiatric patients. This tool becomes the most widely used assessment tool for assessing cognitive impairment. Later, as the head of the department of child psychiatry at New England Medical Center, Dr. Folstein served as the principal investigator of the Collaborative Linkage Study of Autism, a collaborative effort to conduct research on the genetics of autism through the assessment of families with two or more family members with autism. In 2004, Dr. Susan Folstein retired from active academic work but continued to play a significant role in the field of autism as an expert witness in court cases involving the vaccine autism controversy.

Eric Fombonne (b. 1954)

Dr. Fombonne was born and educated in France. He did not first intend to study medicine, but engineering instead. In an interest "to have an impact on people" he switched to medicine, but found that medical school "wasn't enough of a challenge" and so became involved in research as well. He served in the French military in the West Indies, and upon his return to France he led a groundbreaking epidemiological study of psychiatric disorders in children. During this study, he became interested in autism and continued his work in France conducting treatment research in autism. He then spent a sabbatical year working with Michael Rutter and accepted an offer to remain in London at the Institute of Psychiatry as a senior research scientist. There he began his research investigating the proposed relationship between vaccines and autism and assessing the prevalence rates of autism. He has continued his research in these arenas in his position as director of psychiatry at McGill University's Montreal Children's Hospital, which he accepted in 2001. His research has repeatedly indicated that there is no link between vaccines and autism and he is passionate about this line of work. Fombonne has strongly expressed his concern of the repercussions of parents deciding not to vaccinate their children for fear of vaccines causing autism. He took a stance to make his research findings accessible to the public and this mission is summarized by his statement, "Children were dying because fewer vaccines were being given and parents had forgotten that measles can be a killer. It became obvious that scientific evidence had to be communicated efficiently for this debate to be resolved."

Uta Frith (b. 1941)

Dr. Uta Frith was born in Germany and was lured away from studying art history in college to pursue study in experimental psychology in the early 1960s in Saarbrucken, Germany. In 1964 she continued her studies in clinical psychology at the University of London's Institute of Psychiatry and received her PhD in 1968. She took a position at the Medical Research Council where she received mentoring from Lorna Wing and Sir Michael Rutter. Later she was a founding member of the Institute of Cognitive Neuroscience at University College, London. She is credited for transforming developmental psychology into developmental cognitive neuroscience through her careful scientific study of early development, cognition and the disorders of autism and dyslexia. In the field of autism she, along with Simon Baron-Cohen and Alan Leslie, pioneered the exploration of cognitive deficits in autism identifying impairments in mentalizing and central coherence. She has published more than 200 scientific articles, has written and edited a half dozen books, one of which, 1989's *Autism: Explaining the Enigma*, has been translated into 10 languages. She was awarded the prestigious Lifetime Achievement Award by the International Society for Autism Research in 2007.

Daniel Geschwind (b. 1960)

Daniel Geschwind, MD, PhD, is the director of the UCLA Center for Autism Research and Treatment, the Gordon and Virginia MacDonald Distinguished Chair in Human Genetics, director of the Neurogenetics Program, and a professor of neurology and psychiatry at UCLA. He holds a BA from Dartmouth College and received his MD and PhD at Yale School of Medicine before completing his internship, residency, and post-doctoral work at UCLA. Initially a student working toward a chemistry degree, he veered from science to make and star in ski movies in France before training as a neurologist. Later, he turned to study genetics to answer complicated questions regarding social development and communication. With a bibliography of over 130 empirical articles focusing on genetics and neuroscience, Dr. Geschwind has considerably advanced the understanding of the etiology of autism and complex human behavior by addressing the complex questions regarding the genetic basis of autism. In 2001 he joined forces with other researchers affiliated with Cure Autism Now, and together they created the Autism Genetic Research Exchange (AGRE) through which dozens of studies exploring the genetics of autism have been conducted. Through groundbreaking studies he has identified several genomic regions related to autism as well as a specific gene associated with autism and language impairments in males.

Temple Grandin (b. 1947)

Temple Grandin, PhD, is a renowned speaker and author providing insight into the experience of living with autism. Her descriptions are especially powerful given that she herself was diagnosed with autism as a young child in 1950. At the time, her parents were told that she would have to be institutionalized for the rest of her life. However, Dr. Grandin has made the extraordinary transition from not speaking until three and a half years of age (communicating instead by humming and screaming) to eloquently describing her sensory and day-to-day experience as an individual with autism. She is often considered to be one of the most well-known individuals with autism in the world. Dr. Grandin is dedicated to increasing autism awareness in the national and international community and has given countless talks and lectures across the United States and in other countries. She has also been featured on several major television programs, including a documentary about her life. Dr. Grandin's books elegantly describe her perception of the world and her views on social interactions. Titles include *Thinking in Pictures* and *The Way I See It*.

Dr. Grandin's profession is actually a designer of livestock handling facilities and the majority of facilities across the country use Dr. Grandin's designs. She is a professor of animal science at Colorado State University and is a strong advocate for utilizing humane practices in the slaughtering of livestock. Dr. Grandin obtained her BA at Franklin Pierce College, her MS in animal science at Arizona State University, and her PhD in animal science from the University of Illinois in 1989. A film starring Claire Danes was recently released documenting Dr. Grandin's early life, school years, and career beginnings as an animal scientist.

Stanley Greenspan (b. 1941)

Stanley Greenspan, MD, is a psychiatrist and psychoanalyst who developed a popular autism intervention called Floortime. Dr. Greenspan attended Harvard University for his undergraduate work and received his medical degree from Yale Medical School in 1966. He is currently a clinical Professor of Psychiatry and Pediatrics at George Washington University Medical School and Chairman of the Interdisciplinary Council on Developmental and Learning Disorders. His Floortime method is a form of play therapy utilizing social interactions and relationships to teach children with developmental delays, including autism. Floortime operates within a framework of capitalizing on a child's emotions and interests to create learning opportunities. In Floortime following the child's lead and natural interests are essential in challenging the child toward skill mastery. The interactions and methods are often viewed by parents, clinicians, and children to be fun and enjoyable experiences. With younger children, these playful interactions generally occur on the "floor," but, as children age, naturalistic teaching opportunities grow to include more advanced social experiences, such as conversations and interactions in other settings. Emphasis is placed on the role of parents because of the importance of their emotional relationships with the child. Floortime is often used as a complementary treatment to other more structured behavioral interventions, such as Applied Behavior Analysis. Dr. Greenspan continues to conduct trainings and workshops in Floortime methods and training DVDs are available on his Web site.

Portia Iversen (dates unknown) and Jonathan Shestack (b. 1959)

Portia Iversen, an Emmy Award–winning art director and writer, and Jonathan Shestack, a film producer, founded a nonprofit research foundation and parent advocacy organization called Cure Autism Now (CAN) in 1995. The Los Angeles–based couple learned that their son, Dov, was diagnosed with severe autism and were unsatisfied with the limited resources and research on autism that was going on at that time. Their discontent sparked a strong desire to help move the field forward quickly and Iversen and Shestack established CAN to encourage progress toward the goal of raising funds to support autism research and increase attention to the disorder. They lobbied countless groups, from private individuals to congress, for funds to put toward autism research. CAN went on to raise $10 million per year for autism research. Many autism scientists have credited this organization with changing the face of autism because of the attention and funding that it brought to the disorder.

Soon after establishing CAN, Iversen and Shestack cofounded the Autism Genetics Resource Exchange (AGRE) in 1997, which is the world's largest gene bank open to the scientific community to help search for genetic influences in autism. Portia Iversen established the International Meeting for Autism Research (IMFAR) in 2000, which is an annual conference specific to autism research. She also has published a book describing her son's life entitled *Strange Son* as well as a number of scientific research articles on autism genetics and neural functioning in autism.

In 2007, CAN merged with Autism Speaks (another nonprofit parent-founded organization) to become the primary autism parent advocacy organization and research foundation in the world. Iversen and Shestack continue to be involved in the Autism Speaks foundation and Iversen serves on the advisory board.

Leo Kanner (1894–1981)

Leo Kanner was born in Austria, studied in Berlin until World War I, at which point he entered military service. Following the war he returned and finished his medical education at the University of Berlin. In 1921 he received his MD degree. In 1924 he emigrated to the United States and took a position as an assistant physician in South Dakota. Six years later, he was invited to develop and head the first child psychiatry division at the pediatric hospital of Johns Hopkins University. He remained Director of Child Psychiatry at Johns Hopkins until he retired in 1959. In 1935, he published the first book of child psychiatry written in English. Dr. Kanner is credited for first describing autism in his case reports of 11 children with a pattern of disorders marked by significant impairments in social interactions, delays in language and odd use of communication, and restricted interests and repetitive behaviors. In this pioneering 1943 publication, he reports that several children demonstrating this pattern of behaviors had come to his attention since 1938. In his paper, he reflects on Dr. Bleuler's use of the word *autism* and so titles his manuscript "Autistic Disturbances of Affective Contact."

Ami Klin (b. 1960)

Ami Klin, PhD, is another well-known autism researcher. Dr. Klin is the Director of the Autism Program at the Yale Child Study Center and is an Associate Professor of Child Psychology and Psychiatry at Yale University. He received his BA at the Hebrew University of Jerusalem in 1983 and his PhD in Psychology at the University of London in 1988. Dr. Klin's research has provided insight into the neural mechanisms of socialization and their disruption in autism.

Dr. Klin is particularly well known for using novel methods to study and track social processes in individuals with autism. For instance, Dr. Klin often uses eye-tracking technology in which sensors detect the direction of eye gaze and match it onto an object of reference in an individual's visual field. Eye-tracking studies provide insight into the processes of visual scanning and allow us to infer what individuals are attending to and, perhaps, what draws their interest in their environment. Results from Dr. Klin's studies suggest that individuals with autism track and attend to different elements of naturalistic social interactions and situations as compared to typical peers. An important finding from Dr. Klin's laboratory was that individuals with autism tend to look at an individual's mouth when they are talking rather than at their eyes and often focus on details in a room rather than people involved in an emotional social exchange.

Robert and Lynn Koegel (dates unknown)

Drs. Robert and Lynn Koegel are autism treatment researchers who developed an intervention called Pivotal Response Training (PRT) that is based on the principles of applied behavior analysis. Together, they founded and direct the University of California Santa Barbara Koegel Autism Center that serves as both a research institution and service provider. Dr. Robert Koegel trained at UCLA with Ivar Lovaas, PhD, in the 1970s and 1980s and worked with him on the Lovaas Young Autism Project. Dr. Koegel noted the lack of emotional connectedness and joy shown by the children in the projects, even when they successfully accomplished tasks and learned skills. After leaving UCLA, Dr. Koegel decided to embark on a mission to develop his own behavioral intervention using a child's own motivations and interests as the medium through which intervention is delivered. Natural reinforcers are used instead of tangible, often unrelated rewards. For example, instead of earning a potato chip for correctly pointing to a named color, the child would be rewarded with the opportunity to draw with the color crayon that he/she had correctly named. The rationale behind such techniques is that these teaching moments use a child's own motivation to create a naturally reinforcing learning environment in which acquired skills are more likely to generalize to other settings.

Unlike other ABA programs that focus on one particular skill area at a time, PRT targets multiple "pivotal areas" of a child's development and promote child motivation through strategies such as child choice, task variation, and rewarding efforts to complete a task. The Koegels have been strong advocates of nonaversive strategies in implementing their treatment program and Positive Behavior Support (PBS) is their primary behavior change mechanism.

Karen (b. 1954) and Eric (b. 1952) London

A similar story to that of Portia Iversen and Jonathan Shestack transpired on the East Coast of the United States in the early 1990s. Karen and Eric London's son, Zachary, was diagnosed with autism. His parents were frustrated with, in their perspective, a lack of research being conducted on autism at the time. Consequently, the London's cofounded the National Alliance for Autism Research (NAAR) in 1994. Karen London sacrificed her career as a lawyer to devote her life to her son and helping NAAR move forward with the mission of funding autism research projects. Eric London is a psychiatrist by trade and is known for being in strong opposition to the claim that the disorder is caused by mercury-containing vaccines.

An additional important contribution from the London's was the development of the autism tissue program in NAAR to collect postmortem brains from autism patients and their family members. This program allows scientists to search for chemical, cellular, and anatomical features involved in the underlying neural mechanisms in autism. NAAR's primary means of raising money were organizing walkathons and by the time of its final year as an independent organization, it had committed approximately $30 million to autism research. In 2006, one year before Cure Autism Now (another parent-founded autism organization), NAAR merged with Autism Speaks. The NAAR Autism Tissue Program has continued through Autism Speaks and the London's served on the scientific advisory board of Autism Speaks from 2006 through 2009. In 2009, the couple left the organization stating that they disagreed with Autism Speaks' continued support of research examining the potential of a link between autism and vaccinations in rare cases.

Catherine Lord (b. 1950)

Catherine Lord, PhD, is a world-renowned autism researcher and is currently the director of the University of Michigan Autism and Communication Disorders Center (UMACC), the interim director of the New York University Child Study Center Asperger Institute, and a Professor of Psychology and Psychiatry at the University of Michigan. Dr. Lord is Chair of the Board of Directors for the Simons Foundation and also the Early Intervention in Autism Committee at the National Academy of Science. Dr. Lord did her undergraduate work at UCLA and received her PhD in psychology and social relations from Harvard University. Dr. Lord has published more than a hundred journal articles in addition to books and book chapters and has worked at several universities in her academic career, including the University of North Carolina, University of Minnesota, University of Alberta, Harvard University, and University of Chicago.

Dr. Lord is particularly well known for the development of several tools that are widely used during diagnostic evaluations of autism. The Autism Diagnostic Observation Schedule (ADOS) is a standardized means for clinicians and researchers to quantify and assess autism-related symptoms. The Autism Diagnostic Interview (ADI) is a semistructured parent interview designed to document developmental history of autism symptoms as well as current strengths and challenges. The ADOS and ADI are now considered gold-standard diagnostic tools in assessing autism and are used throughout the world to help diagnose autism.

Dr. Lord's research has centered on following young children with autism through early childhood, into adolescence, and now through adulthood. She is the first to provide a truly developmental perspective of the disorder throughout the course of the lifetime. In addition to her academic achievements, Dr. Lord is known for her devotion to the betterment of individuals with autism and her sharp clinical acumen in working with families affected by autism.

O. (Ole) Ivar Lovaas (b. 1927)

Dr. Lovaas is considered by many as the father of applied behavioral analysis and the first to demonstrate the effectiveness of behavioral intervention for the treatment of autism. He grew up in Norway and moved to the United States on a scholarship to Luther College in Iowa. As a professor of psychology at the University of California—Los Angeles, Dr. Lovaas applied the principles of behaviorism that indicate that behavior is guided and shaped through the rewarding of desirable behaviors and the punishment of undesirable behaviors to the treatment of autism. In a 1965 article in *Life* magazine, "Screams, Slaps & Love: A Surprising, Shocking Treatment Helps Far-gone Mental Cripples," his treatment method received considerable attention. In his initial studies, Dr. Lovaas used "aversives" essentially physical punishment to direct behavior in addition to using rewards. In later incarnations of the ABA-based treatment technique, sometimes referred to as discrete trial training, "aversives" were discontinued and only rewards utilized to shape behavior. Although the etiology of autism was still under considerable debate at the time of his initial treatment studies, Dr. Lovaas eschewed the principle of identifying the cause to define the treatment and said, "you have to put the fire out first before you worry how it started." Following the publication of his 1987 paper demonstrating the effectiveness of the treatment through scientific analysis, Dr. Bernard Rimland wrote an editorial for Autism Research Institute's newsletter in which he stated, "when the history of autism is written, the name of Ivar Lovaas will be writ far larger than the names of his many short sighted critics."

Peter Mundy (dates unknown)

Peter Mundy, PhD, is a clinical and developmental psychologist and a prominent autism researcher. He currently is the Lisa Capps Professor of Neurodevelopmental Disorders and Education at the University of California, Davis School of Education, and serves as the director of educational research at the M.I.N.D. Institute. Prior to his current position, Dr. Mundy was a long-standing professor of psychology at the University of Miami. He is the founding director of the University of Miami Center for Autism and Related Disabilities and the founding co-director of the Marino Autism Research Institute at Vanderbilt University. Dr. Mundy obtained his BA in psychology at Stockton State College, New Jersey in 1976, and his MS in 1979 and PhD in 1981 in developmental psychology from the University of Miami.

Dr. Mundy's main area of focus has been in joint attention and social cognition in autism. He has published over a hundred scholarly articles and book chapters. His early work with Dr. Marian Sigman contributed to an understanding that joint attention impairments may be a fundamental component of social challenges in autism. Dr. Mundy's work in this area has helped propagate the field toward earlier identification and diagnosis of autism. Diagnostic tools and early intervention now often focus on joint attention skills in autism, partly due to Dr. Mundy's research efforts. In his more recent work, Dr. Mundy has conducted longitudinal studies of the development of joint attention in typical children. He reports that individual differences in infant joint attention predict social outcomes and social competence in typically developing children.

Isabelle Rapin (dates unknown)

Isabelle Rapin, MD was born in Lausanne, Switzerland, and from the age of 10, she knew that she wanted to be a physician. She was one of a dozen women that attended the Lausanne medical school from which she graduated in 1952. Following graduation, Dr. Rapin moved to New York City where she completed her residency and focused on child neurology. She accepted a position at Albert Einstein College of Medicine in 1958, shortly after the school was founded. Once there she became a prolific scientist, educator, and practitioner, publishing more than 200 articles and books since the 1950's and helping countless families and children with autism. Dr. Rapin began her career interested in language and communication disorders in childhood and studied auditory processing in the brain. Her career later shifted to a focus on autism spectrum disorders. Among other areas within the field of autism, Dr. Rapin's research has largely involved the presentation of a variety of language-based disorders in autism, the neurobiology of autism and, more recently, on the subtyping and classification of autism.

She was a founding member of the Child Neurology Society and the International Child Neurology Association and served in the American Academy of Neurology and American Neurological Association. She has been honored with Autism Society of America's award for excellence in autism research and the Lifetime Achievement Award from the International Society for Autism

Research. She has also provided advice for newcomers to the field of medicine, "Consider every patient a potential source of new knowledge, describe what you see, pursue your interests vigorously, and learn to cut corners and prioritize. Find a good mentor, enjoy what you do, and be lucky."

Bernard Rimland (1928–2006)

Dr. Rimland is best known for his long time advocacy for individuals with autism and for challenging the "refrigerator mother" theory of autism. Born in the Midwest, he moved to Southern California at 12 years of age, and in the late 1920s, he attended college at San Diego State University. He subsequently traveled to the University of Pennsylvania to complete a doctoral degree in experimental psychology in 1953. He returned to southern California and took a position with the navy following the completion of his PhD. His son, Mark, was born three years later and subsequently diagnosed with autism. During Mark's early years, the predominant theory regarding the cause of autism was that poor, cold, unloving parenting led to autism. Dr. Rimland spoke out against this cause, most notably in his book published in 1964: *Infantile Autism: the Syndrome and It's Implications for a Neural Theory of Behavior*. Shortly thereafter, Dr. Rimland joined forces with other parents at a meeting he organized in New Jersey and set the groundwork for the establishment of the parent organization: the Autism Society of America. Two years later, he founded the Autism Research Institute with a mission to conduct and foster research to improve diagnosis, treatment, and prevention of autism. He is credited with initially championing that autism is a neurodevelopmental disorder and more recently attributed as first espousing the notion of an autism epidemic and the idea that mercury in vaccines play a causal role in autism. Upon his death at the age of 78, countless obituaries reported that the father of modern autism research had died.

Edward Ritvo (dates unknown)

Edward Ritvo, MD, is child psychiatrist and professor emeritus at the UCLA School of Medicine. He joined the medical school faculty at UCLA in 1963 and decided to, as he says in his book

Understanding the Nature of Autism and Asperger's Disorder, "set out to slay the fire-breathing dragon we called at that time 'atypical autistic ego development' . . . and have been jousting with this same mean dragon ever since." Dr. Ritvo has been a pioneer in the field of autism and Asperger's Disorder. He is the author of more than 100 scientific papers on autism and Asperger's syndrome and has published several books on autism, including *Understanding the Nature of Autism and Asperger's Disorder* and a storybook about autism called *Joey and Sam: A Heartwarming Storybook About Autism, a Family, and a Brother's Love.*

Dr. Ritvo's research in the 1970s focused on autism diagnosis and identification of milder forms of the disorder and spectrum of challenges involved in autism. Later in his career, Dr. Ritvo was part the UCLA–University of Utah epidemiologic survey of autism and published findings of an important twin study reporting monozygotic concordance rates for autism of 95.7 percent compared to 23.5 percent in dizygotic twins. Dr. Ritvo coauthored the official diagnostic criteria for ASD in the *Diagnostic and Statistical Manual of Mental Disorders.* He has been a strong opponent of the alleged "autism epidemic," instead citing improved ability to detect milder forms of the disorder as being responsible for the increased rates of diagnosis. Dr. Ritvo earned the Lifetime Achievement Award from the International Society for Autism Research in 2010.

Sally Rogers (b. 1948)

Sally Rogers, PhD, is a developmental psychologist who is best known for her work in autism treatment and interventions. She received her doctoral degree in developmental psychology with a specialization in intellectual and developmental disabilities, and is currently a professor of psychiatry and behavior science at the M.I.N.D. Institute at University of California Davis Medical Center. She received her BA from Ashland College in 1969 and PhD from Ohio State University in 1975. Dr. Rogers and her colleagues developed an internationally known intervention designed to promote social interactions and language development in children with autism called the Denver Model (so named because Dr. Rogers was working at the University of Colorado Health Sciences Center at the time it was developed). Dr. Rogers is also the director of the Collaborative Programs of Excellence in Autism Research (CPEA) at the M.I.N.D. Institute and is an active clinician. She continues to be involved in diagnostic evaluations and provides treatment to families in addition to running her research studies.

Although the Denver Model overlaps some with the traditional behavioral approach pioneered by psychologists such as Ivar Lovaas, PhD, the Denver Model utilizes more of a developmental perspective and alternates between intensive teaching trials and developing social-communicative skills through more naturalistic means. Dr. Rogers asserts that these skills are best taught and learned within the context of social relationships, so great emphasis is placed on learning and understanding through emotional exchanges between people. The Denver Model has been applied both in home therapy programs, center-based treatments, and within school environments. More recently, Dr. Rogers collaborated with researchers at the University of Washington, including Geraldine Dawson, PhD, to adapt the Denver Model for use with toddlers with autism (called the Early Start Denver Model) in the first randomized, control trial of early intensive intervention in autism. Compared to those receiving intervention available in the community, young children who received the Early Start Denver Model showed significant improvements in IQ, adaptive behavior, and autism diagnosis.

Sir Michael Rutter (b. 1933)

Professor Sir Michael Rutter is considered by many to be the father of child psychology and psychiatry. He completed his basic medical education at the University of Birmingham and 10 years later, in 1965, he accepted an academic post at the Institute of Psychiatry at King's College in London. At the institute he advanced in rank becoming Professor of Child Psychiatry and then Head of the Department of Child and Adolescent Psychiatry. Starting in 1966 he also served as consultant psychiatrist at Maudsley Hospital. He established the Medical Research Council Child Psychiatry Research Unit in 1984 and the Social, Genetic, and Developmental Psychiatry Research Centre in 1994, serving as honorary director of both until 1998. Professor Sir Michael Rutter's research interests have spanned development from childhood to adulthood, childhood resiliency to stressors, the social aspect of schools, dyslexia, infantile autism, antisocial behavior, the effects of deprivation on Romanian orphan adoptees, antisocial behavior, and has spanned the domains of psychiatric epidemiology, psychiatric genetics, and neuropsychiatry. He made significant contributions to understanding development by following the Romanian orphans adopted into Britain in a major study examining the effects of severe early deprivation. His pioneering work in autism included publishing the first population-based twin study with Susan Folstein in 1977 as well as the establishment of diagnostic tools with Catherine Lord and others. In these areas of research he has published more than 40 books as well 400 scientific articles and book chapters. He has received numerous awards including the prestigious Helmut Horten Award in 1997 for his contributions to the clinical practice of autism, the Lifetime Achievement Award from the International Society for Autism Research in 2002, as well as knighthood in 1992.

Eric Schopler (1927–2006)

Psychologist Eric Schopler pioneered the inclusion of parents in treatment of autism as well as the experimental analysis of interventions. He was born in Germany in 1927 and although he reports not being a personal victim of the prevailing anti-Semitism of the day, his father, a prominent lawyer, was encouraged to leave with his family in 1938 for their safety. Eric's family left immediately for the United States where Eric finished high school, joined the U.S. Army, and then attended the University of Chicago. He continued there to receive a graduate degree in social service administration and then a PhD in clinical child psychology in 1964. While a graduate student in Chicago, the young Schopler questioned the notion that autism was caused by rejecting parents and was convinced that through scientific inquiry he could demonstrate the error of this thinking. He approached Bruno Bettelheim, one of the leading authorities on autism of the day, for assistance in conducting empirical research with children with autism. Dr. Bettelheim rejected his ideas and efforts, but Schopler was not deterred from his goal. He took a faculty position at the University of North Carolina where he began a five-year study examining the impact of structured treatment environments on autism symptoms and parent personality characteristics. After completing the study, his treatment modifications were so well received and the children responded so positively that the parents involved in the study petitioned the state to acquire permanent funding. The funding was granted and in 1972, Division TEACCH (Treatment and Education of Autistic and related Communication-handicapped Children) opens its doors in 1972. Dr. Schopler tirelessly continued his work as an editor of the *Journal of Autism and Developmental Disorders* for 24 years, as the director of Division TEACCH, and as a researcher, publishing more than 200 books and research articles before his death at the age of 79.

Robert Schultz (dates unknown)

Robert Schultz, PhD, is the director of the Center for Autism Research (CAR) and the Developmental Neuroimaging Laboratory at Children's Hospital of Philadelphia, and holds an endowed chair in the Department of Pediatrics. As an executive board member and past president of the International Society for Autism Research (INSAR), and scientific advisor for Autism Speaks and the United Kingdom's MRC Neuroimaging Consortium on Autism, Dr. Schultz is actively engaged in the autism research community. Dr. Schultz's own considerable contributions to the understanding of autism come from his groundbreaking imaging research into the brain regions involved in social interactions. By using structural and functional imaging he has gained insights into the processes underlying social interactions, such as face processing, and has published over 100 articles and chapters in the field of psychology and neuroscience. He received his BS from the University of Delaware and his PhD in clinical psychology with a focus on neuropsychology from the University of Texas–Austin.

Marian Sigman (dates unknown)

Dr. Sigman has conducted research in the field of autism for more than 25 years at the University of California in Los Angeles. She joined the faculty at UCLA in 1977 after a move west from Boston University where she received her PhD in 1970. At UCLA she holds faculty appointments in the Department of Psychology and Department of Psychiatry and Biobehavioral Sciences. She was the first president of the International Society for Autism Research, held the position of Chair for the Advisory Committee of the National Childcare Study, and was the founding president for the International Society for Infant Studies. She served as the UCLA director for the Collaborative Program of Excellence (CPEA) in

Autism and the Center for Autism Research and Treatment, one of the NIMH funded Studies to Advance Autism Research and Treatment (STAART) centers. Both the CPEA and STAART collaborations are federally funded centers to conduct research in autism and provide opportunities for collaboration and enhanced data collection to spur scientific findings.

During her tenure at UCLA, Dr. Sigman has authored more than 200 scientific articles and chapters and several books. Dr. Sigman's research has included infant attention (particularly social attention) and its relation to later development and developmental challenges. She is one of the pioneers of the study of a concept called "joint attention" in autism, which involves an individual's ability to attend to an object or event by means of a social partner's eye gaze and/or gesture. Joint attention is crucial to a young child's cognitive, linguistic, and social development and is significantly impaired in young children with autism. It is now considered by some to be one of the earliest expressions of the fundamental impairment in autism. Dr. Sigman's work largely influenced this view. Her more recent research has expanded to include multidisciplinary work involving treatment, genetics, and neurobiology of autism as well as the expression of subthreshold symptoms in infant siblings of children with autism. In 2009, Dr. Sigman received the Lifetime Achievement Award from the International Society for Autism Research.

Marilyn (dates unknown) and Jim (b. 1938) Simons

As was the case for a number of private foundations funding autism research, Jim and Marilyn Simons have a personal attachment to the disorder: their daughter was diagnosed with autism. However, unlike other founders of autism advocacy organizations, autism is only one of the areas of focus for Jim and Marilyn Simons' organization the Simons Foundation. A renowned mathematician by trade, Dr. Jim Simons became independently wealthy through the development of equations used in hedge funds and has donated a large percentage of his wealth to philanthropic causes, including basic science and math research. The Simons' do not often step out into the limelight, but are known for being very involved in the projects that are funded through their foundation.

In 2003, Jim and Marilyn Simons decided to embark on a new initiative for the Simons Foundation and called well-known minds in autism research together in a "Panel on Autism Research" to determine the most important next steps in the field. Since then, the Simons Foundation had dedicated more than $100 million to autism research, primarily through the Simons Simplex Collection (SSC) Project, which is an international, multi-site study examining the genetic causes of autism. The Simons Foundation plans on dedicating many more funds to autism research through the Simons Foundation Autism Research Initiative (SFARI).

Ruth C. Sullivan (b. 1924)

Dr. Sullivan's involvement in the field of autism began in 1963 when her three-year-old child Joseph, her fifth of seven children, was diagnosed with autism. The reigning theory at the time was that cold, aloof mothers were the cause of autism. Dr. Sullivan, a public health nurse, knew that to be untrue and joined forces with Dr. Bernard Rimland and other parents to form what is now known as the Autism Society of America (ASA). She served as the organization's first president. In the years following her son's diagnosis and involvement in ASA, she became an outspoken activist for rights for individuals with disabilities and was instrumental in the passage of the 1975 Individuals with Disabilities Education Act. The act ensures a free public education to all children, including those with disabilities. Four years later she focused her efforts at providing opportunities for adults with autism. She founded the Autism Services Center, which provides group home situations for adults with autism that allow the residents to remain engaged in life. She also played a role in the development of the Autism Training Center at Marshall University and served as a consultant for the movie *Rain Man*. Dustin Hoffman worked with her son during his preparation for his role.

Helen Tager-Flusberg (b. 1951)

Helen Tager-Flusberg, PhD, is a Professor of Anatomy and Neurobiology and Psychology at Boston University and the Director and Principal Investigator at the Lab of Cognitive Neuroscience at Boston University. She did her undergraduate work in psychology at University College, University of London in England and obtained her doctorate degree in Experimental Psychology from Harvard University in 1978. Prior to her current professorship at Boston University beginning in 2001, Dr. Tager-Flusberg was a Professor of Psychology at the University of Massachusetts at Boston where she had been a member of the faculty since earning her doctorate degree in 1978. Dr. Tager-Flusberg's research involves language and social-cognitive development within various populations, especially autism. She also has studied other groups with such genetically based disorders as Williams Syndrome and specific language disorders and is currently researching social cognition in Williams Syndrome. Dr. Tager-Flusberg is known for using a variety of methodologies to answer her research questions, including behavioral tracking and brain imaging. More current autism research of Dr. Tager-Flusberg's has explored the interrelation of genetic, neurological, and cognitive/behavioral functioning in individuals with autism throughout their lifespan. She serves on the editorial board of several professional journals, including the *Journal of Autism and Developmental Disorders* and *Applied Psycholinguistics*. Dr. Tager-Flusberg has published four books on autism spectrum disorders and related fields and written many research articles focusing on linguistic development in children with autism and theory of mind tasks in this population.

Fred Volkmar (b. 1950)

Dr. Fred Volkmar is the director of the Yale Child Study Center, the Irving B. Harris Professor of Child Psychiatry, Pediatrics and Psychology at the Yale University School of Medicine and is Chief of Child Psychiatry at the Yale Children's Hospital. As an active physician focusing on autism research and treatment, he has served on a variety of national and international committees, including the committee on Pervasive Developmental Disorders for the *Diagnostic and Statistical Manual of Mental Disorders*. He is the editor of the *Journal of Autism and Developmental Disabilities* and has published several hundred scientific articles and book chapters. His research in autism focuses on elucidating the nature and various expressions of the fundamental social difficulties in autism. Dr. Volkmar uses innovative techniques to answer his research questions, including functional and structural magnetic resonance imaging, genetic methodologies, and eye tracking technology. His studies using eye tracking (i.e., tracking the movement of individuals' eyes as they watch a monitor or potentially live scenes) revealed that individuals with autism tend to look at nonsocial aspects of a social scene. For example, they may focus on a light switch in a corner of a room rather than on individuals in the center of the room who are having an emotional exchange. Dr. Volkmar has studied individuals with autism of a variety of ages and levels of functioning, with more recent studies of infant siblings of children with autism. He has also written a number of influential books in the field of autism including *Asperger's Syndrome*, *Health Care for Children on the Autism Spectrum*, and *The Handbook of Autism*. Dr. Volkmar is a graduate of the University of Illinois and attended medical school at Stanford University where he received his MD and a master's degree in psychology in 1976.

Lorna Wing (b. 1928)

Lorna Wing, MD, is now a retired British psychiatrist who has been actively involved in the field of autism for more than 40 years and was originally drawn into the area because she has a daughter with autism. Dr. Wing and her colleague Dr. Judith Gould are credited with introducing the concept of the *autism spectrum*, which has changed the face of research and clinical understanding of autism. Her description of variable symptom presentations and severities in autism was in disagreement with Leo Kanner's original 1943 assertion that autism presented as a single entity. Dr. Wing has published numerous journal articles and books describing various symptoms presentations and profiles on the autism spectrum throughout her academic career. She has developed a number of methods for subtyping individuals with autism and developed rating scales to better do so. More recently, Dr. Wing has researched changes in autism prevalence rates and examined possible reasons for this phenomenon, including differences in diagnostic criteria.

Dr. Wing also familiarized the autism world with the research of Hans Asperger, who in the 1940's described a group of high functioning individuals with autistic features. His work went largely unrecognized until Dr. Wing published her academic paper "Asperger's Syndrome: A Clinical Account" in 1981. This clinical account introduced the term *Asperger's Syndrome*, which has been included in the most recent editions of the *DSM*. Together with other parents of children with autism, she founded the National Autistic Society (NAS) in the United Kingdom in 1962. Dr. Wing received a lifetime achievement award from the International Society of Autism Research in 2005 for her significant accomplishments to the field of autism in her career.

Suzanne (b. 1946) and Bob (b. 1943) Wright

Like many of the other important contributors in the field of autism, Bob and Suzanne Wright learned that a family member was diagnosed with autism (a grandson, Christian, in their case) and were compelled to do what they could to help. Their mission was to raise awareness about autism and build upon research into its causes and treatment. The Wrights established the foundation Autism Speaks in 2005 in an effort to achieve this goal. Bob Wright, former CEO of NBC, encouraged colleagues and friends to donate funds to Autism Speaks and raised millions of dollars for autism advocacy. They have raised several hundred million to date and ceaselessly lobbied congress to allocate research money to autism. The couple played a primary role in the successful passage of the Combating Autism Act from which nearly $1 billion in federal funding was dedicated to "autism screening, education, early intervention, prompt referrals for treatment and services, and research."

The Wright's commitment to introducing autism awareness to the global scene encouraged the United Nation to place autism on the global health agenda. After combining forces with other parent-led foundations, including Cure Autism Now, the National Alliance for Autism Research, and Autism Coalition for Research and Education, Autism Speaks is the nation's leading nonprofit organization devoted to autism and a leader in the world in autism advocacy. Additional projects for the Wright's have included the production the short film *Autism Everyday* with the goal of providing a real-life documentary of the stresses (and joys) in the lives of parents and children with autism. This video received national attention and is available in short form on the Autism Speaks Web site.

6

Data and Documents

This chapter focusing on data and documents relevant to ASDs will include information relevant to the characterization and diagnosis of the disorder, screening and early identification processes, neuroscience, prevalence, and intervention.

Domains of Autism

Autism spectrum disorders (ASDs) are defined by behaviorally observed impairments in three domains. These domains include the social domain, the communication domain, and a third behavioral domain focusing on restricted or repetitive interests or behaviors. Examples of impairment in the social domain include atypical use of nonverbal behaviors (such as eye contact or facial expressions) in social interactions, difficulties in establishing or maintaining friendships, a lack of emotional or social reciprocity, and a lack of showing, sharing or giving. Examples of impairment in the communication domain include language delay, deficits in conversational skills, or the use of stereotypic (repetitive) or other atypical speech patterns. Examples in the behavioral domain include the presence of unusual interests, difficulties with transitions, or repetitive motor mannerisms. As Figure 6.1 demonstrates, it is the interaction of impairments in the domains that results in an autism spectrum disorder.

Pervasive Developmental Disorders Umbrella Term

ASDs fall under the category of Pervasive Developmental Disorders in the fourth edition of the Diagnostic and Statistical Manual (DSM-IV;

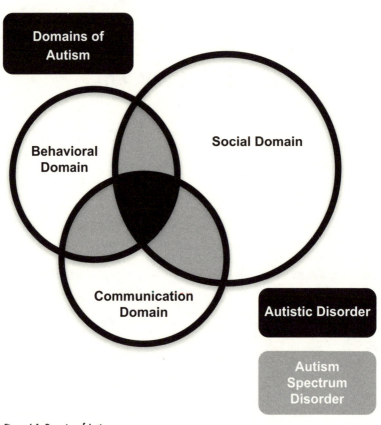

Figure 6.1. Domains of Autism

Source: R. Bernier. 2005. *Autism 101 Lecture.* Reprinted with permission of author.

American Psychological Association 2000). As an umbrella term Pervasive Developmental Disorders are characterized by severe and pervasive impairments in many aspects of an individual's life, including social interactions, communication skills, and presence of stereotyped behaviors. As indicated in Figure 6.2, two other diagnoses, Rett's Disorder and Childhood Disintegrative Disorder, fall into this category of clinical disorders but are themselves not considered part of the autism spectrum.

To meet diagnostic criteria for Autistic Disorder, an individual must demonstrate qualitative impairments in the social, communication, and behavioral domains that results in adaptive functioning in school, home or the community. Further, these impairments must be evident by 3 years of age. This differs from the diagnostic criteria for Asperger's Disorder in that individuals with Asperger's Disorder do not demonstrate any clinically significant language or cognitive delays. More subtle differences between both disorders concern the focus of the behavioral concerns. While in Autistic Disorder the behavioral concerns often focus on repetitive motor mannerisms, difficulties with transitions, ritualized behavior, and preoccupations with parts of objects, in Asperger's Disorder the behavioral concerns are more often marked by interests of markedly unusual intensity that form the focus of learning and conversational topics for the individual with the disorder. Similar to Autistic Disorder, the impairments in the social and behavioral domains must cause clinically significant impairment in social, occupational or other important areas of functioning to warrant a diagnosis. The third diagnostic category under the umbrella term of Autism Spectrum Disorders is Pervasive Developmental Disorder—Not Otherwise Specified (PDD-NOS). This diagnosis is appropriate when an individual demonstrates clinically significant impairments in the social domain along with deficits in either communication or behavior, but when the specific criteria for Autistic Disorder or Asperger's Disorder are not met. For example, this diagnostic category might be appropriate for individuals demonstrating a later age of onset, who have an atypical presentation of symptoms, or who have symptoms that are subthreshold for Autistic Disorder or Asperger's Disorder.

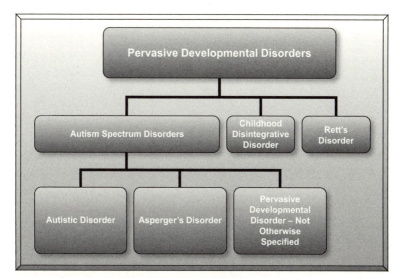

Figure 6.2. The Pervasive Developmental Disorders Umbrella Term

Source: R. Bernier. 2005. *Autism 101 Lecture.* Reprinted with permission of author.

Diagnostic Criteria for Autism Spectrum Disorders

The specific criteria for the diagnosis of ASDs, including Autistic Disorder, Asperger's Disorder, and PDD-NOS are outlined in DSM-IV. First published by the American Psychiatric Association in 1952, the DSM is in its fourth edition, and workgroups are currently working on the next version, with plans for the DSM-V to be released in 2012. Each disorder is given a code following a coding system that corresponds to the International Statistical Classification of Diseases, 10th edition (ICD-10). The text below outlines the diagnostic criteria for the three disorders considered ASDs.
Diagnostic Criteria for Autistic Disorder 299.00

A. A total of six (or more) items from (1), (2), and (3), with at least two from (1), and one each from (2) and (3):

(1) qualitative impairment in social interaction, as manifested by at least two of the following:

(a) marked impairment in the use of multiple nonverbal behaviors such as eye-to-eye gaze, facial expression, body postures, and gestures to regulate social interaction
(b) failure to develop peer relationships appropriate to developmental level
(c) a lack of spontaneous seeking to share enjoyment, interests, or achievements with other people (e.g., by a lack of showing, bringing, or pointing out objects of interest)
(d) lack of social or emotional reciprocity

(2) qualitative impairments in communication as manifested by at least one of the following:

(a) delay in, or total lack of, the development of spoken language (not accompanied by an attempt to compensate through alternative modes of communication such as gesture or mime)?
(b) in individuals with adequate speech, marked impairment in the ability to initiate or sustain a conversation with others?

(c) stereotyped and repetitive use of language or idiosyncratic language?

(d) lack of varied, spontaneous make-believe play or social imitative play appropriate to developmental level

(3) restricted repetitive and stereotyped patterns of behavior, interests and activities, as manifested by at least two of the following:

(a) encompassing preoccupation with one or more stereotyped and restricted patterns of interest that is abnormal either in intensity or focus

(b) apparently inflexible adherence to specific, nonfunctional routines or rituals?

(c) stereotyped and repetitive motor mannerisms (e.g., hand or finger flapping or twisting, or complex whole-body movements)?

(d) persistent preoccupation with parts of objects

B. Delays or abnormal functioning in at least one of the following areas, with onset prior to age 3 years: (1) social interaction, (2) language as used in social communication, or (3) symbolic or imaginative play.

C. The disturbance is not better accounted for by Rett's Disorder or Childhood Disintegrative Disorder.

Diagnostic Criteria for Asperger's Disorder 299.80

A. Qualitative impairment in social interaction, as manifested by at least two of the following:

(1) marked impairment in the use of multiple nonverbal behaviors such as eye-to-eye gaze, facial expression, body posture, and gestures to regulate social interaction

(2) failure to develop peer relationships appropriate to developmental level

(3) a lack of spontaneous seeking to share enjoyment, interest or achievements with other people, (e.g., by a lack of showing, bringing, or pointing out objects of interest to other people)

(4) lack of social or emotional reciprocity

B. Restricted repetitive & stereotyped patterns of behavior, interests and activities, as manifested by at least one of the following:

   (1) encompassing preoccupation with one or more stereotyped and restricted patterns of interest that is abnormal either in intensity or focus
   (2) apparently inflexible adherence to specific, nonfunctional routines or rituals
   (3) stereotyped and repetitive motor mannerisms (e.g., hand or finger flapping or twisting, or complex whole-body movements)
   (4) persistent preoccupation with parts of objects

C. The disturbance causes clinically significant impairments in social, occupational, or other important areas of functioning.
D. There is no clinically significant general delay in language (e.g., single words used by age 2 years, communicative phrases used by age 3 years).
E. There is no clinically significant delay in cognitive development or in the development of age-appropriate self help skills, adaptive behavior (other than in social interaction) and curiosity about the environment in childhood.
F. Criteria are not met for another specific Pervasive Developmental Disorder or Schizophrenia.

Pervasive Developmental Disorder Not Otherwise Specified (Including Atypical Autism) 299.80
This category should be used when there is a severe and pervasive impairment in the development of reciprocal social interaction or verbal and nonverbal communication skills, or when stereotyped behavior, interests, and activities are present, but the criteria are not met for a specific Pervasive Developmental Disorder, Schizophrenia, Schizotypal Personality Disorder, or Avoidant Personality Disorder. For example, this category includes "atypical autism"—presentations that do not meet the criteria for Autistic Disorder because of late age of onset, atypical symptomatology, or subthreshold symptomatology, or all of these.

Constellation of Symptoms in an Individual with ASD

While many symptoms are common to individuals with ASD, each individual with ASD is unique. In order to meet diagnostic criteria for an ASD, it is not necessary to have all symptoms in each domain. For example, in order to meet diagnostic criteria for Autistic Disorder, an individual must demonstrate qualitative impairment in two of four possible areas in the social domain, in two of four possible areas in the communication domain, and at least one of four possible areas in the behavioral domain, with a minimum of six areas of impairments across all three domains. Figure 6.3 demonstrates a possible constellation of symptoms for an individual with an ASD. Another child with an ASD, while still meeting diagnostic criteria for an ASD, may demonstrate a completely different constellation of symptoms.

This heterogeneity in symptom presentation is complicated by additional factors such as cognitive ability that can vary even within the diagnosis of Autistic Disorder. That is, one individual with Autistic Disorder could have an IQ well above average, while another individual may have an IQ indicating intellectual disability (formerly called mental retardation). This range is pronounced throughout the ASDs. While cognitive ability varies widely in ASD, with some individuals demonstrating above average IQ, approximately one-third to one-half of individuals with ASD also have intellectual disability (Autism and Developmental Disabilities Monitoring Network Surveillance year 2002 Principal Investigators 2007). Intellectual functioning in its own right significantly impacts an individual's functioning. This could profoundly impact the presentation for an individual with autism. For example, two individuals with ASD with a similar constellation of social, communicative, and behavioral impairments could radically differ in intellectual functioning, one individual having intellectual disability while the second individual displays above average cognitive skills. This disparity in intellectual functioning could result in radically different presentations. Further, individuals with similar constellations of symptoms may also have radically different developmental trajectories with one child with ASD responding well to intervention while a second child continues to demonstrate significant impairments despite a myriad of attempted treatments.

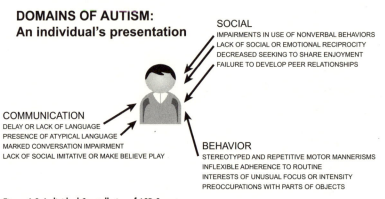

DOMAINS OF AUTISM:
An individual's presentation

SOCIAL
IMPAIRMENTS IN USE OF NONVERBAL BEHAVIORS
LACK OF SOCIAL OR EMOTIONAL RECIPROCITY
DECREASED SEEKING TO SHARE ENJOYMENT
FAILURE TO DEVELOP PEER RELATIONSHIPS

COMMUNICATION
DELAY OR LACK OF LANGUAGE
PRESENCE OF ATYPICAL LANGUAGE
MARKED CONVERSATION IMPAIRMENT
LACK OF SOCIAL IMITATIVE OR MAKE BELIEVE PLAY

BEHAVIOR
STEREOTYPED AND REPETITIVE MOTOR MANNERISMS
INFLEXIBLE ADHERENCE TO ROUTINE
INTERESTS OF UNUSUAL FOCUS OR INTENSITY
PREOCCUPATIONS WITH PARTS OF OBJECTS

Figure 6.3. Individual Constellation of ASD Symptoms

Source: Based on R. Bernier, J. Winter, and J. Varley. 2008. *My Next Steps: A Parent's Guide to Understanding Autism.* Seattle, WA: University of Washington Autism Center

Screening for Autism Spectrum Disorders

Red Flags for the Identification of Autism

In 1999 the Child Neurology Society and American Academy of Neurology proposed to establish practice parameters regarding the screening and identification of autism. A multidisciplinary committee led by Dr. Pauline Filipek was tasked with reviewing what was currently known about the identification and diagnosis of autism to develop these practice parameters. Following a systematic review of more than 2,500 published articles, the multidisciplinary consensus committee, composed of representatives from nine professional organizations, four parent-based organizations, and representatives from the National Institutes for Health, published the practice parameters. In the published manuscript, the panel reviewed the findings in the literature, proposed two levels of screening and identification, and outlined the process for evaluation at both levels. The panel also identified parental concerns that constitute important red flags for autism in each of the three behavioral domains of autism and established those that warranted immediate evaluation.

The two levels of screening and evaluation consist of a first level to be performed on all children at well-child visits and used to detect any aspect of atypical development. During this screening primary care providers, through standardized questionnaire and parent interview, would conduct a quick screening for any evidence of atypical development, not necessarily autism. Based on this initial broad screen, if indicated the provider should conduct specific level-one testing, such as audiological or lead-poisoning testing or the administration of autism specific standardized question-

naires. If the outcome of this level-one screening indicates the possibility of autism, then the provider would make a referral to a provider with autism expertise for level-two screening. The second level of the screening process focuses specifically on the diagnostic evaluation and assessment of autism. For this level the panel proposed an in-depth process that includes: (1) referral to early intervention or school district; (2) formal diagnostic procedures by experienced clinician based on DSM-IV criteria; (3) comprehensive evaluation to determine profile and inform treatment recommendations including (a) expanded medical and neurologic evaluation; (b) speech-language-communication evaluation; (c) cognitive evaluation; (d) adaptive behavior evaluation; (e) sensorimotor and occupational therapy evaluation; (f) neuropsychological, behavioral, and academic evaluation; g. assessment of family functioning and resources; and (h) expanded laboratory evaluation as needed focusing on metabolic testing, genetic testing, electrophysiologic testing, and neuroimaging (for features not explained by diagnosis of autism).

The identified parental concerns that constitute red flags that are suggestive of further level-one screening and potentially level-two screening as well as those behaviors that warrant immediate diagnostic evaluation (at level two) are identified below.

Concerns Presented by Parents that Are Red Flags for Autism
*Adapted from Filipek et al. 2000

Communication Concerns

Child does not respond to his/her name

Child's language is delayed

Child does not follow instructions

Child appears deaf at times; seems to hear sometimes but not others

Child does not point or wave goodbye

Child has a loss of any language

Child cannot tell parents what he/she wants

Social Concerns

Child does not smile socially

Child prefers to play alone

Child is very independent; gets things for him/herself; does things early

Child has poor eye contact

Child seems to be in his/her own world

Child tunes others out

Child is not interested in other children

Behavioral Concerns

Child has tantrums

Child does not know how to play with toys

Child gets stuck on things over and over; perseverates on things

Child toe walks

Child has unusual attachment to objects (i.e., is always holding a certain object)

Child lines things up (i.e., cars, chalk, pens, etc.)

Child is oversensitive to certain sounds or textures

Child has odd movement patterns

Child is hyperactive/uncooperative or oppositional

Further Developmental Evaluation Is Absolutely Indicated If:

Child is not babbling by 12 months

Child is not gesturing (pointing, waving bye-bye, etc.) by 12 months

Child has no single words by 16 months

Child has no spontaneous two-word phrases by 24 months

Child has a loss of any language or social skills at any age

Source: Based on Filipek, P., Accardo, P., Ashwal, S., Baranek, G., Cook, E., Dawson, G., Gordon, B., Gravel, J., Johnson, C., Kallen, R., Levy, S., Minshew, N., Ozonoff, S., Prizant, B., Rapin, I., Rogers, S., Stone, W.,

Teplin, S., Tuchman, R., Volkmar, F. 2000. "Practice Parameter: Screening and Diagnosis of Autism: Report of the Quality Standards Subcommittee of the American Academy of Neurology and the Child Neurology Society." *Neurology* 55 (4): 468–79.

Neuroscience of Autism Spectrum Disorders

Social Brain Systems Impaired in ASD

There are several theories regarding the neurological pathology of ASD. Two of these theories have received support as a result of productive exploration of brain structures relevant to social information processing and the interconnectivity among these brain regions. Given the predominance of social dysfunction in the clinical presentation of ASD, the primacy of social behavior in human development, and the cross-species evolutionary conservation of brain systems apparently evolved to regulate interactions with others of the same species, social brain theories posit that (a) specific human brain systems exist to process information pertaining to other humans (Brothers 1990) and (b) autistic dysfunction originates in these brain systems, exerting secondary, peripheral impacts through developmental effects. For example, one proposed hypothesis, the social motivation hypothesis, suggests that reduced social drive leads an individual with ASD to pay less attention to people which results in the consequent failure of developmental specialization in brain systems that rely upon experience to fully develop, such as processing information from faces (Dawson, Webb, and McPartland 2005).

Interconnectivity theories, in contrast to social information processing theories, have predominantly focused on nonspecific brain processes, in which the nature of the information processed is relevant only insofar as it requires distributed brain function. For example, it has been posited that, due to poor long range connectivity in the brains of individuals with ASD, simple, local processing is intact while complex, distributed information processing is impaired in ASD (Minshew and Williams 2007). Given the complexity of social interaction, functioning of distributed brain structures is required for rapid and easy processing of social information. According to connectivity theories, it is a disruption in connectivity that impairs social processing, not dysfunctional brain systems specific to social information processing. Evidence for atypical interconnectivity in ASD derives primarily from studies of brain structure (Barnea-Goraly et al. 2004), fMRI (Kleinhans et al. 2008), and EEG coherence (Murias et al. 2007), and, to date, has focused primarily on functional connectivity, or the temporal correlation between neural activity in separate brain areas.

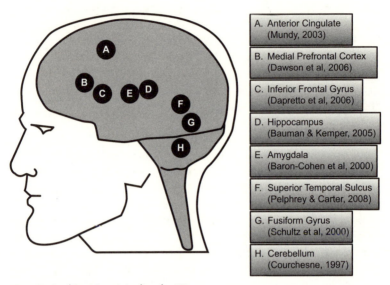

Figure 6.4. Social Brain Circuitry Implicated in ASD

Source: Bernier, R. 2002. *Neuroscience of Autism Lecture.* Reprinted with permission of author.

The social information processing theory suggests that the impairments observed in autism are the result of dysfunctional circuitry related to brain structures relevant to processing social information. Figure 6.4 highlights some brain structures and systems related to social information processing that have been implicated in ASD.

Face Perception in Autism

The ability to rapidly and easily process information in the human face is an early developing and essential skill for social interaction. Very young infants demonstrate a preference for faces and objects that look like faces and will attend to longer and look at faces (Goren, Sarty, and Wu 1975; Johnson et al. 1991). Further, young infants can use information from faces. For example, infants only days old are able to remember their mother's face (Bushnell, Sai, and Mullin 1989) and infants as young as 42 minutes old demonstrate the ability to imitate facial expressions (Meltzoff and Moore 1977). This early attentional preference and ability to use information from faces from very early on, provides infants with valuable *information about the world around them. Through faces, humans learn about emotions, communication, and the intentions of others.*

Researchers have learned about the perception of faces at the behavioral, anatomical, and neurophysiological level. Face perception abilities become specialized within the first months of life (de Haan, Johnson, and Halit 2003; Leppanen and Nelson 2009) and continue to develop over childhood such that children move from processing faces using feature-based strategies to using more holistic, configural processing strategies. That is, when looking at a car one might notice the headlights, the fenders, and the emblem on the hood to determine what kind of car it is. This would be using a feature-based processing strategy, as opposed to a holistic strategy that humans rely upon for face processing (Farah, Tanaka, and Drain 1995).

Advances in technology have allowed researchers to understand the brain systems involved in the perception and processing of faces and information from faces. Imaging research using positron emission tomography (PET) and functional magnetic resonance imaging (fMRI) indicate that when looking at faces, a region of the occipitotemporal cortex in the brain, the fusiform gyrus, is activated (Haxby et al. 1994; Kanwisher, McDermott, and Chun 1997; Puce et al. 1995). Studies using electrophysiology have also provided insight into face processing. Using event-related potentials (ERPs), changes in the brain's electrical activity in response to a specific event that are recorded via sensors attached to the scalp, scientists have shown a negative going peak in the brain's electrical activity that occurs approximately 170 milliseconds after perceiving a face. This peak is termed the N170, as it is a negative going wave that peaks around 170 milliseconds after the event (Bentin et al. 1996). The use of electrophysiology, which has a much finer temporal resolution that fMRI, on the order of milliseconds as opposed to seconds, provides insight into the speed at which information from faces is processed in the brain.

Research on face processing in autism indicates that this is a specific area of social interaction that is impacted in autism. At the behavioral level, infants who later go on to be diagnosed with autism attend to faces less than typically developing children or children with intellectual disability (Osterling and Dawson 1994) and perform more poorly at tests of face and emotion recognition (Hobson 1986). Further, individuals with autism attend differently to faces. While typically developing individuals attend more to eyes, individuals with autism focus more on the mouth than on the eyes (Klin et al. 2002). At the neurological level, it has been shown that individuals with autism show less activation of the traditional face processing region of the brain, the fusiform gyrus, than typical individuals (Schultz et al. 2000). Further, research employing electrophysiological measurement and assessment of the N170 has shown that individuals with autism show delays in processing faces (McPartland et al. 2004).

Dr. McPartland and colleagues compared the ERP component, the N170, in response to pictures of faces in a group of adults with autism and a same age group of comparison adults with typical development. They found that the participants with autism showed a longer N170 latency, the characteristic N170 peak was delayed, compared to the comparison group. Importantly, they found that the electrophysiological delay correlated with behavioral measures of face recognition. Figure 6.5 shows the ERP waveform for both the group of participants with autism (in black) and the comparison group (in gray). The negative going peak is highlighted in gray and demonstrates that this peak is delayed in the individuals with autism. While the delay is on the order of milliseconds, at the brain level this is significant. One could imagine that if processing faces takes longer, even just moments longer, it delays the processing of all the other information related to faces or could lead to a mismatch in connecting information from faces and other information in the social world, such as language or context. This underscores the importance of face processing in social interac-

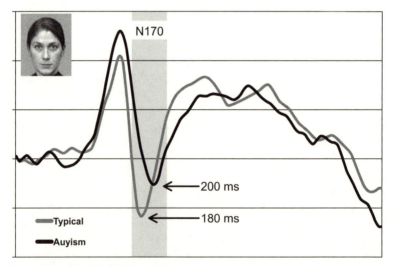

Figure 6.5. Face Perception in Autism

Source: Based on J. McPartland, G. Dawson, S. Webb, H. Panagiotides, and L. Carver. 2004. "Event-related Brain Potentials Reveal Anomalies in Temporal Processing of Faces in Autism Spectrum Disorder." *Child Psychology and Psychiatry* 45:1235–45. Reprinted with permission of author.

tion and the potential importance of face processing to the cascade of social impairments in autism.

Prevalence of Autism Spectrum Disorders

Prevalence Estimates from Educational Records

Prevalence is defined as the number of cases of a given disorder in the population at a given time. Although studies to determine the prevalence of autism began shortly after Leo Kanner first reported on the disorder, interest was kindled early in the 21st century following reports of increasing numbers of children with ASD being treated in the school systems across the United States. Reviews of educational records from the late 1990s and early 2000s has indicated that there is an increasing number of children being diagnosed with ASDs in the United States (Gurney et al. 2003; Newschafer et al. 2005). Moreover, the data from these records most likely underestimates the number of children with a diagnosis of ASD because children may receive special education services for difficulties other than ASD, such as speech therapy.

A rich source of data of this sort comes from information concerning children with disabilities who are served under the Individuals with

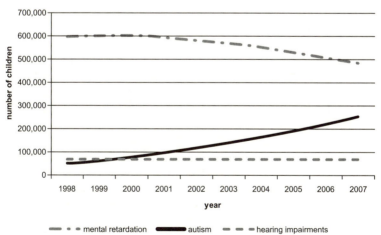

Figure 6.6. Number of Children Served under the Individuals with Disabilities Education Act

Source: Based on data available at http://www.ideadata.org.

Disabilities Education Act (IDEA). The IDEA is a federal law, established in 1990, that provides guidelines of special education and early intervention service provision by state and public agencies. The data that are collected indicates the number of children being served under the federal act for a given IDEA disability category (e.g., autism or hearing impairment) across all 50 states. Based upon IDEA data, Figure 6.6 shows the number of children being served by the IDEA between the years of 1998 and 2007 for three disability categories: mental retardation, hearing impairment, and autism. The graph shows the rising number of children being served falling into the IDEA category of autism, the decreasing number of children being served falling under the label of mental retardation, and the relatively consistent number of children with hearing impairment being served over the 10-year span.

Prevalence Estimates from Monitoring Networks

Data from educational records provide an important perspective on treatment and services usage for children with disabilities, but are not the best indicators of the true prevalence of the disorder. Special education records provide information about numbers of children receiving special education services with a given disorder, but this is not the same as the number of children with a given disorder. More importantly, the eligibility criteria for determining which disability category a child falls into varies state by state and these criteria do not map precisely onto the diagnostic criteria as established by the medical community for all states. For example, in order to establish eligibility for receiving services for autism in the state of Washington a child requires a diagnosis from a professional, licensed provider following the criteria outlined in DSM-IV. This is not the case for all states, and while IDEA states that the eligibility criteria cannot be any more restrictive than these criteria, the criteria can be looser.

This suggests that the accurate determination of prevalence rates must be achieved through different means. Accurate estimates of prevalence are critical because it allows for the comparison of rates across differing time points or populations. The characteristics of individuals with a disorder, such as race or gender, can be identified and this can help guide research to determine causes as well as risk and protective factors.

In an attempt to address this need to accurately estimate the prevalence of ASDs in the United States, the Centers for Disease Control formed the collaborative network, the Autism and Developmental Disabilities Monitoring (ADDM) Network. The ADDM network, consisting initially

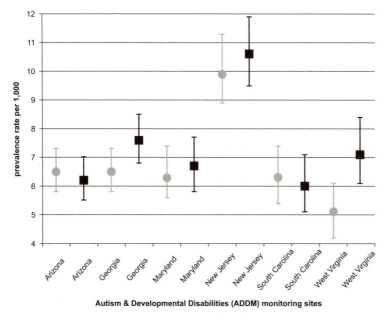

Figure 6.7. Prevalence of ASD in 8-year-old Children in 2000 and 2002 in Six States Participating in the Autism and Developmental Disabilities Monitoring (ADDM) Network

Source: Based on data presented by Autism and Developmental Disabilities Monitoring (ADDM) Network in *Morbidity and Mortality Weekly Report, Surveillance Summaries,* February 9, 2007, 56 (SS01): 1–11 and 12–28.

of sites in 6 states and expanded to include 17 states, utilizes standardized measures to accurately count the number of eight-year-old children with an ASD in each project area.

The ADDM network established the prevalence rates for ASD in 2000 for 6 states and in 2002 for 17 states. The overall prevalence rate across the six included states for 2000 was 6.7 per 1,000 eight-year-old children, which is approximately 1 in 150 children. The rate in 2002 was very similar at 6.6 per 1,000 eight-year-old children, which roughly approximates to 1 in 150 children as well. Based on data from the six states involved in both estimates, the results indicate that the prevalence rate of ASD was relatively stable in Arizona, Maryland, New Jersey, and South Carolina, but increased in Georgia and West Virginia. Interestingly, in 2000 only 70 percent, and in 2002 only 61 percent, of the identified children with ASDs in Maryland were receiving special education services.

*This suggests that if educational records were utilized to estimate preva-
lence rates, the rate would be an underestimate. Figure 6.7 shows the prevalence rates for the six participating ADDM sites during both the 2000
and 2002 assessments. The figure also shows that prevalence rates differed
by state, with the rate of New Jersey falling above the rates obtained for the
other states.*

Ethnic Differences in Prevalence of Autism Spectrum Disorders

*Although prevalence estimates across countries and within the United
States suggest that autism affects members of all race and ethnicities
equally, some research suggests there are differences in patterns of diagnosis of autism between racial groups. White Medicaid-eligible children with
autism in Philadelphia county receive a diagnosis about one and a half
years, on average, earlier than African-American children and two and a
half years earlier than Latino children (Mandell, Listerud, Levy, & Pinto-
Martin, 2002). Additionally, African American children with ASD were
nearly 3 times more likely than White children to be diagnosed with another
disorder prior to receiving a diagnosis of ASD (Mandell, Ittenbach, Levy,
and Pinto-Martin 2007). According to data presented in the Department
of Education's 2001 IDEA report, students in the United States identified
as African American or Asian/Pacific Islander were served by the IDEA
under the category of ASD at twice the rate of those who were American
Indian/Alaskan or Hispanic (Dyches, Wilder, and Obiakor 2001).*

*A study to estimate ASD prevalence in the United States reported
findings by racial group (Kogan et al. 2009). To conduct this study questions regarding autism were included in the 2007 National Survey of
Children's Health (NSCH) conducted by the Centers for Disease Control
and Prevention's National Center for Health Statistics. The NSCH is a
telephone survey of child health and well-being and is used as a representative sample of all of the United States. To estimate the prevalence of
ASD and assess differences in prevalence rates by racial group, the authors
asked parents participating in the survey if the child under discussion had
ever been diagnosed with autism. Of 77,911 children between the ages of
3 and 17, 911 had reportedly been diagnosed with autism at some point
during their lives. This yields a population estimate of 110 per 10,000
children having a diagnosis of ASD and representing approximately
673,000 children in the United States (Kogan et al. 2009). In regards to
race and ethnicity, the authors of the study found that non-Hispanic, black*

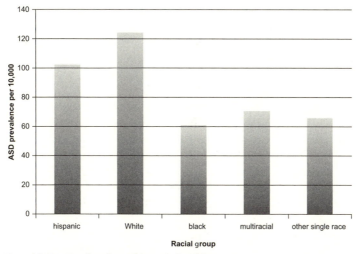

Figure 6.8. Point Prevalence Rates of Autism by Racial Group

Source: Based on data presented in M. Kogan, et al. 2009. "Prevalence of Parent-Reported Diagnosis of Autism Spectrum Disorder Among Children in the US, 2007." *Pediatrics* 124: 1395–403.

children had 57 percent lower odds of having an ASD diagnosis than non-Hispanic, white children. Non-Hispanic, multiracial and non-Hispanic other single race (not black or white) children both had 42 percent lower odds of having an ASD diagnosis than non-Hispanic, White children (Kogan et al. 2009). As shown in Figure 6.8, there were no differences in prevalence rates for Hispanic or white children, and this finding differed from previous research, but the authors note that there is evidence to suggest that in Hispanic households in which Spanish is the primary language the prevalence of an ASD diagnosis is lower than that found in this study.

Interventions in Autism Spectrum Disorders

Treatment and Interventions for Autism Spectrum Disorders

The vast array of treatments and interventions that are used or have been used to treat individuals with autism ranges from education-based treatments to animal-based treatments to pharmacological intervention. The large number and diversity of interventions available to families is staggering and can be overwhelming for many families just receiving a diagnosis.

The interventions for autism fall into three main categories: psychoeducational, psychopharmacological, and complementary (Charman and Clare 2004). There are currently no interventions that cure autism, few have been rigorously assessed by the scientific community, few have been found to demonstrate improvement of symptoms, and some interventions have even proven harmful.

However, within the psychoeducational domain, interventions based on applied behavioral analysis (ABA) have been shown to be effective in providing long-term benefits through well-controlled studies (Howlin, Magiati, and Charman 2009). Studies of behaviorally based interventions have demonstrated gains in intellectual ability and symptom reduction for individuals with autism. Although there is no direct evidence that intervention begun earlier has a greater benefit than intervention begun later, consensus among the scientific community is that children with autism should begin a behaviorally based intervention program as early as possible (Dawson and Zanolli 2007). A perceived drawback for many families is that these early, intensive behavioral interventions (also known as EIBI) are costly and time consuming.

A number of medications falling in the psychopharmacological category have been used to treat children and adults with autism. However, the focus of treatment with pharmacological agents has been on improving symptoms associated with autism, but not the core social communicative deficits. Medications have been used to ameliorate associated attentional deficits, depression, anxiety, sleep problems, obsessive compulsions or rituals, as well as self-injurious or repetitive behaviors and tics. Although there are many conflicting results in the research literature, support has been found for the effectiveness of medication to reduce depression, repetitive behaviors, hyperactivity and aggression in autism (Charman and Clare 2004).

A third category of interventions focuses on complementary or alternative treatments. These treatments are labeled alternative because they currently fall outside what is considered mainstream provision of care and are sometimes termed Complementary and Alternative Medicine (CAM) treatments. Into this category falls the collection of treatments called biomedical treatments. The majority of these treatments have not been rigorously studied using well-designed research studies. Most of the studies that have been conducted assessing these interventions lack sufficient experimental controls, suffer from small sample sizes, and have resulted in findings that have not been replicated in independent studies. Some treatments, including secretin and facilitated communication, have been demonstrated to have no effectiveness, while other treatments have yielded potentially promising initial findings that require rigorous evaluation and *replication (Myers, Johnson, & American Academy of Pediatrics Council on Children With Disabilities 2007).*

The list of interventions identified below includes most of the treatments and interventions that are used or have been used to treat individuals with autism. The presence of a treatment or intervention on the list does not mean that there is any scientific evidence for its effectiveness. Importantly, the Treatments and Interventions table below is not in any way an endorsement of the listed treatments.

Treatments and Interventions for Autism Distributed by Category

Psycho-Educational

Standard

ART THERAPY

MUSIC THERAPY

PLAY THERAPY

OCCUPATIONAL THERAPY

SPEECH THERAPY

PROMPT SPEECH THERAPY

PHYSICAL THERAPY

Behavioral Interventions

APPLIED BEHAVIORAL ANALYSIS

EARLY START DENVER MODEL

PIVOTAL RESPONSE TRAINING

DISCRETE TRIAL TRAINING

SOCIAL STORIES

SOCIAL SKILLS TRAINING

SOCIAL GROUPS

INTEGRATED PLAY THERAPY

Educational and Integrated Services

TEACCH

DAILY LIFE THERAPY

Technology Based

VIDEO MODELING

Alternative and Augmentative Communication

VISUAL SCHEDULES

PICTURE EXCHANGE COMMUNICATION SYSTEM
(PECS)

COMPLEMENTARY

Animal Based

CANINE COMPANION

DOLPHIN THERAPY

HIPPOTHERAPY

THERAPEUTIC HORSEBACK RIDING

Spirituality Based

PRAYER

ENERGY HEALING

Diets and Supplements

DIETARY INTERVENTION (E.G., GLUTEN-FREE,
CASEIN-FREE DIET [GFCF DIET]; YEAST FREE;
KETOGENIC)

HOMEOPATHY

IMMUNOTHERAPY

VITAMIN THERAPY

SECRETIN

MELATONIN

Medical Procedures

CHELATION

HYPERBARIC OXYGEN THERAPY

ELECTROCONVULSIVE THERAPY

Relationship-Based Interventions

FLOORTIME

SON-RISE TREATMENT

GENTLE TEACHING

HOLDING THERAPY

RELATIONSHIP DEVELOPMENT INTERVENTION

PEER MENTORING

Integrated Interventions

LINWOOD METHOD

SCERTS MODEL

Physiological Interventions

CHIROPRACTIC

CRANIO-SACRAL THERAPY

ACUPUNCTURE AND ACUPRESSURE

YOGA

THERAPEUTIC MASSAGE

PATTERNING THERAPIES

MILLER METHOD

AUDITORY INTEGRATION THERAPY

RHYTHMIC ENTRAINMENT INTERVENTION

SAMONAS

SENSORY INTEGRATION THERAPY

TOMATIS METHOD

VISION THERAPY

IRLEN LENS SYSTEM

BIOFEEDBACK AND NEUROFEEDBACK

AQUATIC THERAPY

Technology Based

ASSISTIVE TECHNOLOGY

TEACHTOWN

FAST FORWARD

ONLINE COMMUNITIES

Alternative and Augmentative Communication

FACILITATED COMMUNICATION
RAPID PROMPTING

Psycho-Pharmacological

PHARMACOLOGICAL INTERVENTIONS (INCLUDING:
ANTI-CONVULSANTS; ANTI-DEPRESSANTS; ANTI-
FUNGALS; ANTI-HYPERTENSIVES; ANTI-PSYCHOTICS;
ANXIOLYTICS; MOOD STABILIZERS; SEDATIVES;
STIMULANTS; AMONG OTHERS)

Source: Based upon information in Charman, T., and P. Clare. 2004. *Mapping Autism Research: Identifying UK priorities for the Future.* London: National Autistic Society; and Exhorn, K. S. 2005. *The Autism Sourcebook.* New York: Regan.

Guidelines for Evaluating Interventions

There is a vast array of treatment and intervention options marketed and available to families of children with autism. The list of potential interven-

tion is dizzying and ranges from such empirically supported treatments as ABA-based therapy to treatments that focus on specific areas of difficulty, such as speech therapy for communication difficulties, occupational therapy for motor or sensory concerns, or medication for associated conditions such as depression or seizures. In addition to these treatments supported by the medical community there is an equally dizzying array of treatments termed Complementary and Alternative Medicines (CAMs). These treatments range from chelation, facilitated communication, vitamin supplements, dietary interventions, dolphin therapy, to social skills training, auditory integration, and secretin injections. And the list goes on. With this vast array of options, some of which have scientific support for their effectiveness while others have no scientific support, it is important that families have tools available to aid in the evaluation of these potential intervention options. B. J. Freeman published guidelines in 1997 to provide a framework for families to evaluate intervention programs for autism (Freeman 1997). Freeman highlights that the critical factor to remember when evaluating programs is that every child with autism is unique and what is appropriate for one child with autism may not be appropriate for another and only programs with a goal to "help a person with autism become a fully functioning member of society" are appropriate (Freeman 1997, p. 647).

The selected text below provides the list of general guidelines proposed by B. J. Freeman and the corresponding five questions that must be asked of any program after considering these guidelines.

Guidelines for Evaluating Treatments for Autism

1. Approach any new treatment with hopeful skepticism. Remember the goal of any treatment should be to help the person with autism become a fully functioning member of society.
2. Beware of any program or technique that is touted as effective or desirable for every person with autism.
3. Beware of any program that thwarts individualization and potentially results in harmful program decisions.
4. Be aware that any treatment represents one of several options for a person with autism.
5. Be aware that treatment should always depend on individual assessment information that points to it as an appropriate choice for a particular child.
6. Be aware that no new treatment should be implemented until its proponents can specify assessment procedures necessary to determine whether it will be appropriate for an individual with autism.

7. Be aware that debate over use of various techniques are often reduced to superficial arguments over who is right, moral and ethical and who is a true advocate for the children. This can lead to results that are directly opposite to those intended including impediments to maximizing programs.
8. Be aware that often new treatments have not been validated scientifically.

Questions to Ask Regarding Specific Treatments

1. Will the treatment result in harm to the child?
2. How will failure of the treatment affect my child and family?
3. Has the treatment been validated scientifically?
4. Are there assessment procedures specified?
5. How will the treatment be integrated into the child's current program? Do not become so infatuated with a given treatment that functional curriculum, vocational life and social skills are ignored.

Source: Freeman, B. J. 1997. "Guidelines for Evaluating Intervention Programs for Children with Autism." *Journal of Autism and Developmental Disorders* 27: 641–51. Reprinted with permission from Springer Science + Business Media, © 1997.

Guidelines for Evaluating Complementary and Alternative Treatments

Given the myriad of complementary and alternative medical therapies available to families, physicians are faced with the need to help counsel families in their evaluation of CAMs. In an effort to aid in the assessment of potential malpractice liability issues around CAMs, Cohen and Eisenberg provide a framework in a 2 × 2 design. Through this framework, the authors also provide a framework for counseling families in the evaluation of any CAM. In this design the evaluator's decision about the treatment should be based on available evidence concerning the safety of the treatment and on the effectiveness of the treatment. As shown in Figure 6.9 a

	effectiveness: limited or inconclusive evidence	effectiveness: evidence in support
safety: evidence in Support	Tolerate; caution; closely monitor for effectiveness	Recommend treatment; continue to monitor
safety: limited or inconclusive evidence	Avoid and discourage	Consider tolerating; caution; closely monitor for safety

Figure 6.9. Decision Matrix for Complementary and Alternative Medical Therapies

Source: Based on M. Cohen and D. Eisenberg. 2002. "Potential Physician Malpractice Liability Associated with Complementary and Integrative Medical Therapies." *Annals of Internal Medicine* 136: 596—603.

treatment for which there is evidence in the scientific and medical literature of effectiveness and safety would be recommended while a treatment for which there is no evidence of either, would be avoided and discouraged. A treatment for which there is evidence of safety but for which there is inconclusive evidence of effectiveness could be tolerated but it would be important to advance with caution and its effectiveness would need to be closely monitored. If a treatment's effectiveness was supported in the literature but evidence of its safety was inconclusive, the evaluator could consider tolerating the treatment, but close monitoring and caution would be imperative.

Applied Behavioral Analysis and Discrete Trial Training

Applied Behavioral Analysis (ABA) is a general term that encompasses intervention approaches designed to change behavior based on operant behavioral principles. ABA is based on the concept that behaviors paired or followed by a reward (termed a reinforcer) become more positive and increase, while behaviors paired with or followed by a punishment or negative consequence become more negative and decrease. Treatments based on ABA principles are the only intervention approach that is deemed effective for addressing ASDs. In children with autism, these treatments generally involve an intensive teaching method of carefully reinforcing certain behaviors while ignoring others. Social and communication skills are usually the focus of ABA and skills are generally taught methodically, starting with more foundational skills and moving onto more complex skills. Therapies based on ABA principles are often done in a home setting by trained therapists. Parents can also be taught therapy techniques based on ABA and are often encouraged to use such methods when interacting with their children. A child's ABA-based therapy program is usually designed by a psychologist and is individualized for each child in order to address the child's specific strengths and weaknesses.

There are many different types of ABA-based therapy programs. Discrete Trial Training (DTT), Pivotal Response Training (PRT), and the Early Start Denver Model (ESDM) are just a few of the many behaviorally based interventions available. While all ABA interventions follow the principles of operant conditioning and incorporate data collection and clear progress monitoring, in each distinct treatment program, there are differences in the structure, setting, or focus of the intervention. Some treatments provide naturalistic treatment settings and relate the reward or reinforcement to the skill area being taught to increase the value of the reward in that context. For example, if the focus of a skill training activity is counting, a child might be provided with the option to count an object of interest to him, such as colored blocks or toy cars, and have the opportunity to play with the cars after demonstrating mastery of the counting skill. PRT focuses on two "pivotal" areas of behavior: motivation and responsivity to multiple cues, based on the framework that these two pivotal areas are central to a wide range of functioning and by impacting these two areas, improvements in behavioral functioning will cascade. DTT, another treatment program, is less naturalistic and focuses on breaking down tasks into basic steps and teaching these basic skills on subskill at a time while reducing the number of prompts until the child has mastered the skill.

Dr. Ivar Lovaas, professor of psychology at the University of California in Los Angeles, was an early pioneer of applying the principles of ABA and through initial work demonstrated the effectiveness of Discrete Trial Training in producing gains in cognition and behavior in children with autism (Lovaas 1987). DTT is also called the "Lovaas approach" because Dr. Lovaas popularized this type of instructional strategy in the

1970s and 1980s. A discrete trial in this treatment program is the basic unit of instruction in which there are several distinct behaviorally based components to the instructional routine. The first step is the instruction to which the therapist would like the student to respond, which in behavioral terms is called the discriminative stimulus. The second component, the prompt, is optional and may be unnecessary. The verbal or physical prompt is used to aid in helping the student respond appropriately. The next component is the response and this is what the child does. This is followed by the reward, or reinforcement, and serves to increase the desired response. The final component is an inter-trial interval that differentiates one trial from the next. The student's response, as well as the prompt used, if any, during the trial can be recorded in the inter-trial interval. This will form the data that are used to determine when the child has mastered the skill being trained and when the next skill should be addressed.

Data collection and monitoring is an important facet of ABA-based treatments. The data is used to guide goal development for an individual's treatment program and to monitor improvement. Results from the data can indicate if the treatment program is effective and if not can indicate that the program needs to be modified.

Figure 6.10 shows a typical ABA-based treatment data tracking sheet with sample data included. On the data sheet the skill area of interest (or the discriminative stimulus), the desired response, and the reinforcement that is being used is recorded. For each skill a chart marked by trial number is included so that the therapist can record the student's response as well as any prompt needed for that trial. A key for the abbreviations used in the table is listed at the top of the data sheet to remind the therapist of the response and prompt types to record. Following a cycle of discrete trials, the percentage of correct responses without prompts is calculated.

An example of a discrete trial session that would generate the data in Figure 6.10 follows:

Billy's teacher is working on vocabulary development with him and is focusing on animals given Billy's recent trip to the petting farm. The instructions of the task are to identify the toy cat among the collection of animal toys on the table between them. The discriminative stimulus is "show me the cat" and the expected response is the identification of the cat with a point. Billy's teacher knows that Billy is motivated by verbal praise, but that his favorite snack is a goldfish cracker so, his teacher will use both praise and the goldfish crackers to reinforce responses. Billy's teacher notes the date and time on the sheet (Oct 12th, 9:00 a.m.).

ABA Based Treatment Data Tracking Sheet

Child Name: Billy _____

Prompt types:
V: verbal, PV: partial verbal
M: model, PM: partial model
P: physical, PP: partial physical
Response: C: correct, I: incorrect
NR: no response

Skill/Stimulus: __animals, cat__
Desired Response/Behavior: __point to cat toy__
Reinforcement: __praise and goldfish crackers__
Date/Time: __Oct 2, 9 am__

Trial #:	1	2	3	4	5	6	7	8	9	10	11	12	13	14	15	16	17	18	19	20	21	22	23	24
Response:	NR	NR	NR	-	+	+	-	-	+	+	+	+	+	-	-	+	+	+	+	+				
Prompt:	P	P	P	PP	PP	M	V	V	V	V	PV	V	V	V	PV									
% Correct:	25%																							

Skill/Stimulus: __animals, cat__
Desired Response/Behavior: __point to cat toy__
Reinforcement: __praise and goldfish crackers__
Date/Time: __Oct 3, 9:15 am__

Trial #:	1	2	3	4	5	6	7	8	9	10	11	12	13	14	15	16	17	18	19	20	21	22	23	24
Response:	NR	-	-	+	+	-	+	+	+	+	+	-	+	+	+	-	+	+	+	+				
Prompt:	P	PP	PP	PP	V	V	PV	PV																
% Correct:	50%																							

Skill/Stimulus: __animals, cat__
Desired Response/Behavior: __point to cat toy__
Reinforcement: __praise and goldfish crackers__
Date/Time: __Oct 4, 2 pm__

Trial #:	1	2	3	4	5	6	7	8	9	10	11	12	13	14	15	16	17	18	19	20	21	22	23	24
Response:	-	-	+	+	-	+	+	+	+	-	+	-	+	+	+	+	+	+	+	+				
Prompt:	V	V	PV	PV	PV																			
% Correct:	60%																							

Figure 6.10. Example ABA-based DTT Data Tracking Sheet with Sample Data

Source: R. Bernier. 2004. *Autism Interventions Lecture.* Reprinted with permission of author.

Trial #1

TEACHER: "Show me the cat." [Discriminative Stimulus]

Billy sits at the table but does not make any response. The teacher takes Billy's hand, shapes it so that he is making a pointing gesture, and directs his index finger to the cat. [Prompt & Response]

TEACHER: "Good job. That's the cat!" [Reinforcement]

During the inter-trial interval, the teacher quickly notes on the data sheet that Billy could not identify the cat independently on this trial.

Trial #2

TEACHER: "Show me the cat."

Billy remains seated and maintains fleeting eye contact with his teacher, but does not respond. The teacher waits a few seconds and then again takes Billy's hand, shapes it so that he is making a pointing gesture, and directs his index finger to the cat.

TEACHER: "You got it. That's the cat!"

During the inter-trial interval, the teacher quickly notes on the data sheet that Billy could not identify the cat independently on this trial.

Trial #3

TEACHER: "Billy, show me the cat."

Again, Billy makes no response and after a few seconds, the teacher takes Billy's hand, shapes it so that he is making a pointing gesture, and directs his index finger to the cat.

TEACHER: "Yup. There's the cat!"

During the inter-trial interval, the teacher quickly notes on the data sheet that Billy could not identify the cat independently on this trial.

Trial #4

TEACHER: "Show me the cat, Billy."

The teacher waits a few seconds and then reaches to grab Billy's hand but before touching him, he points to the animal closest to him, the dog.

TEACHER: "That's the dog. This is the cat!" The teacher moves Billy's hand to the cat. "Yup, that's the cat."

During the inter-trial interval, the teacher quickly notes on the data sheet that Billy incorrectly identified the cat independently on this trial following a partial physical prompt.

Trial #5

TEACHER: "Show me the cat, Billy."

The teacher waits a few seconds and then reaches to grab Billy's hand but while reaching toward him, he points to the cat.

TEACHER: "Great job! This is the cat!" The teacher hands Billy a goldfish cracker to increase the reward value for responding to the instruction.

During the inter-trial interval, the teacher quickly notes on the data sheet that Billy correctly identified the cat following a partial physical prompt.

An additional 15 trials are completed during this session. At the completion of the 20 trials, the percentage correct is tallied and for this session Billy's percentage correct is 25%. This is recorded on the data-tracking sheet. The teacher then moves to a different skill to focus on.

Example of Monthly Progress Data Sheet

The detailed data collected during individual sessions can be recorded over a period of time to track progress in an instructional program or skill area. By recording trial-by-trial data and examining the data across time, trends in learning patterns can be identified and incorporated into treatment planning. The data can be used to determine if a student has gained mastery of the skill in question by a simple, quick examination of the data. For example, using Billy's example, Billy's teacher decided that prior to beginning the animal language training program mastery would be de-

Monthly Progress Data Sheet

Child Name: Billy
Skill Area: cat identification
Active/Maintenance? active

Month: October
Mastery Criteria: 100% correct on 3 consecutive days, prompt free

Percent/Date	1	2	3	4	5	6	7	8	9	10	11	12	13	14	15	16	17	18	19	20	21	22	23	24	25	26	27	28	29	30	31
100%																															
90%								X	X																						
80%						X	X	X	X																						
70%					X	X	X	X	X																						
60%				X	X	X	X	X	X																						
50%			X	X	X	X	X	X	X																						
40%			X	X	X	X	X	X	X																						
30%			X	X	X	X	X	X	X																						
20%		X	X	X	X	X	X	X	X																						
10%	X	X	X	X	X	X	X	X	X																						
0%	X	X	X	X	X	X	X	X																							

Skill Area: dog identification
Active/Maintenance? active

Month: October
Mastery Criteria: 100% correct on 3 consecutive days, prompt free

Percent/Date	1	2	3	4	5	6	7	8	9	10	11	12	13	14	15	16	17	18	19	20	21	22	23	24	25	26	27	28	29	30	31
100%									X	X	X																				
90%					X	X	X	X	X	X	X																				
80%				X	X	X	X	X	X	X	X																				
70%				X	X	X	X	X	X	X	X																				
60%			X	X	X	X	X	X	X	X	X																				
50%		X	X	X	X	X	X	X	X	X	X																				
40%		X	X	X	X	X	X	X	X	X	X																				
30%	X	X	X	X	X	X	X	X	X	X	X																				
20%	X	X	X	X	X	X	X	X	X	X	X																				
10%	X	X	X	X	X	X	X	X	X	X	X																				
0%	X	X	X	X	X	X	X	X	X	X	X																				

Figure 6.11. Example ABA-based Treatment Monthly Progress Sheet with Sample Data

Source: R. Bernier. 2004. *Autism Interventions Lecture.* Reprinted with permission of author.

fined as successful independent correct identification of an animal occurring 100 percent of 20 trials for three consecutive days. Using information transferred from a data sheet to a monthly tracking sheet allows Billy's teacher to quickly determine if and when Billy mastered animal identification skills.

Figure 6.11 shows an example of a monthly progress sheet with data from Billy's example. The data from Billy's discrete trials during the month of October (Figure 6.10 shows data collected on October 2nd, 3rd, and 4th) is transferred from data tracking sheets to the monthly progress sheet at the end of each day. The monthly progress sheet demonstrates that it took Billy 10 days to master the identification of cats and that after 3 days his ability in this area improved dramatically but not enough to demonstrate mastery until that 10th day. The example sheet also demonstrates performance in a second skill area, in this case a very similar one, the identification of another animal. This is helpful because the teacher can quickly notice that Billy tends to quickly improve after just a few short days, but struggles to achieve fluency or mastery as defined by the teacher until several days of consistent practice.

Social Stories

There are a number of supportive techniques that can be helpful for individuals with autism. Social stories (or social scripts) are one such technique. A social story is a type of behavioral support. It is a short, developmentally appropriate story that describes a standard routine (e.g., a trip to the doctor's office) from beginning to end. Developmentally appropriate means using terms and concepts that are appropriate for a child's mental age, not chronological age. For example, Sam is an eight-year-old boy with autism who also has cognitive impairments. Cognitive testing estimates that he has an intelligence quotient (IQ) of 50. This means that he is functioning at a mental age of a four-year-old. As a result, terms and concepts that are appropriate for a four-year-old would be more appropriate for Sam than concepts directed at his chronological age. A social story also describes any potential difficulties that may be encountered along the way during an event or day (e.g., "The shot at the doctor might hurt a little, but my mom will be there and it will be alright"). Often social stories include pictures embedded in the text. Many children with autism have difficulties processing long strings of verbal information but many also have strengths in processing visual information. By including pictures in the story and capitalizing on the visual strengths many children with autism possess, comprehension of the social story can be maximized. Social scripts are a type of social story in which the child's behavior or speech is scripted for him or her to help manage the social situation. Ultimately, social stories are designed to help children with autism anticipate future events and to minimize surprises associated with this new event.

The sample social story shows an example of a description of a downhill skiing lesson written at a developmental level for an eight-year-old child.

Today we will learn to ski.

We have to wear a big jacket and helmet when we go skiing.

This is so we stay warm and safe.

Skiing is fun because I get to glide down a hill on the snow.

The wind feels good on my face.

Sometimes I fall down when I learn to ski.

It might hurt a little, but I will stand up and be OK.

I will follow my teacher's directions so she will keep me safe.

Going slowly and not being too close to other people is the safest way to ski.

There will be a lot of grown-ups and kids in line to go on the chairlift.

That's OK because everyone is there to have fun.

Everyone will be proud of me because I had fun when I learned to ski!

Source: Varley, J., and R. Bernier, R. 2007. *Strategies for Working with Individuals with Autism.* Seattle, WA: Presentation for Outdoors for All

Economic Cost of Autism Spectrum Disorders

The economic costs of ASDs in the United States are considerable. For ASDs, the direct medical costs, such as physician services, medication, and hospital visits; direct nonmedical costs, such as special education, respite care, and supported employment services; and indirect costs, which include lost productivity in the workplace, reduced work hours, or departure from the workforce, tally to an estimated $35 billion to treat all the

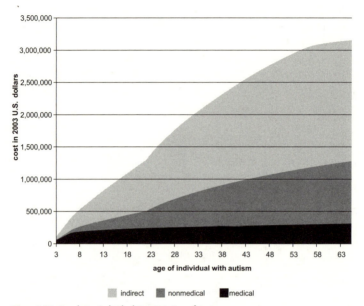

Figure 6.12. Cumulative Individual Economic Cost of Autism

Source: Based on data presented in M. Ganz. 2009. "The Lifetime Distribution of the Incremental Societal Costs of Autism." *Archives of Pediatric and Adolescent Medicine* 161: 343–49.

individuals diagnosed in a year over their lifetimes (Ganz 2006). In a study of health care utilization and costs in California's Kaiser Permanente Medical Care Program, the study authors found that costs for hospitalizations, clinic visits, and medications were more than double for the children with ASD compared to children without ASD (Croen et al. 2006). After adjusting for age and gender the total costs are more than threefold higher for children with ASDs. According to this 2006 study and previous studies (Guevara et al 2003; Newacheck 2005), it is a minority of the children with ASDs who require either psychiatric or non-psychiatric hospitalizations that increase the overall cost. A cost calculation based on data culled from the scientific literature, national databases for health care costs, and labor statistics and databases, resulted in an estimated lifetime cost for an individual with ASD of $3,160,384 combining direct and indirect costs (Ganz 2009). Figure 6.12 graphically demonstrates these data presenting costs in 2003 dollars for an individual diagnosed at age 3. The figure highlights the significant direct medical costs in the first 5 years of life and the decrease in these costs during each year across the lifespan, but with an ever-increasing cumulative tally.

Vaccine Injury Compensation Program and Autism

The vaccine injury compensation program is a federally funded program to provide financial compensation to families following an adverse reaction to vaccination. Through this program started in 1986, families can quickly receive financial compensation of $900,000 in a very short time provided it can be definitively demonstrated that the injury was caused by the vaccination. This program was started to alleviate the number of lawsuits directed against vaccine makers that in the mid-1980s threatened to end vaccine manufacturing. While this program does not entirely protect vaccine makers, because if families are dissatisfied with rulings pharmaceutical companies can be sued in state courts, it has dramatically reduced the number of lawsuits.

Because of the belief that vaccines cause autism (see Chapter 2 for history of this controversy) many families have made claims to the vaccine injury compensation court. Between 1999 and 2007, more than 5,000 families made claims that vaccines caused their child's autism. This number overpowered the vaccine injury compensation court, and as a result the court decided to address the claims like a class-action lawsuit. Called the Omnibus Autism Proceeding, the trial began in the summer of 2007 and focused on three specific cases.

On February 12, 2009, the courts revealed their verdict. After reviewing the testimony concerning the three cases and including expert witnesses from both sides, the three judges that comprise the panel determined that for each case there was no evidence that the children's autism was caused by the MMR vaccine and thimerosal. In the Opinion and Order on the case of Cedillo v. Secretary of Health and Human Services, Judge Wheeler reported that there was no evidence that Michelle Cedillo's autism was caused by the MMR vaccine and thimerosal.

In the United States Court of Federal Claims; No. 98-916V; (Filed: August 6, 2009)

Vaccine Act; Omnibus Autism Proceeding; Effect of Thimerosal and Measles, Mumps, and Rubella Vaccine in Causing Autism; Burden of Proof; Standard of Review; Analysis of Causation-in-Fact Evidence; Assessment of Expert Testimony.

THERESA and MICHAEL CEDILLO, as Parents and Natural Guardians of MICHELLE CEDILLO, Petitioners, v. SECRETARY OF HEALTH AND HUMAN SERVICES, Respondent.

Ronald C. Homer, with whom were *Kevin P. Conway* and *Sylvia Chin-Caplan,* Conway,

Homer & Chin-Caplan, P.C., Boston, Massachusetts, for Petitioners.

Lynn E. Ricciardella, with whom were *Michael F. Hertz*, Acting Assistant Attorney General, *Timothy P. Garren*, Director, *Catharine E. Reeves*, Acting Deputy Director, and *Gabrielle M. Fielding*, Assistant Director, Torts Branch, Civil Division, United States Department of Justice, Washington, D.C., for Respondent.

Opinion and Order

WHEELER, Judge.

This case is before the Court for review of the Special Master's February 12, 2009 decision dismissing Theresa and Michael Cedillo's petition for compensation under the National Childhood Vaccine Injury Act of 1986, 42 U.S.C. § 300aa-1 et seq. (2006) (the "Vaccine Act"). See Cedillo v. Sec'y of HHS, No. 98-916V, 2009 WL 331968, at *1 (Fed. Cl. Spec. Mstr. Feb. 12, 2009) (hereinafter "Cedillo"). Petitioners assert that their daughter, Michelle Cedillo, suffered severe autism and gastrointestinal injuries from various vaccines containing thimerosal, and from the measles, mumps and rubella ("MMR") vaccine. This case was the first of three test cases under the Office of Special Masters' Omnibus Autism Proceeding established in July 2002 to assist in the resolution of approximately 5,000 autism cases pending in this Court. The other two test cases, also decided by Special Masters on February 12, 2009, are Snyder v. Secretary of Health & Human Services, No. 01-162V, 2009 WL 332044 (Fed. Cl. Spec. Mstr. Feb. 12, 2009) and Hazlehurst v. Secretary of Health & Human Services, No. 03-654V, 2009 WL 332258 (Fed. Cl. Spec. Mstr. Feb. 12, 2009), aff'd No. 03-654V, 2009 WL 2371336 (Fed. Cl. July 24, 2009).

In brief summary, Petitioners argue that Michelle Cedillo was a normal child for her first sixteen months until she experienced the effects of eleven vaccinations containing thimerosal, and the MMR vaccination. Pet'r Br. 2, 17 n.41, Mar. 16, 2009. Thimerosal is a compound consisting of mercury and other components that has been used since the 1930s in very small amounts as a preservative in vaccines to prevent fungal and bacterial contamination. Cedillo, at *17. The Cedillos claim that the ethyl mercury in thimerosal and the MMR vaccine damaged their daughter's immune system, and that due to her immune deficiency, she was unable to clear from her body the measles virus contained in the MMR vaccine. Instead, the measles virus persisted and replicated in Michelle's body, causing her to suffer inflammatory bowel disease. The Cedillos also contend that the measles virus ultimately entered Michelle's brain, causing inflammation and autism.

In a 174-page decision, Special Master George Hastings rejected all of Petitioners' contentions, observing that "the evidence was overwhelmingly contrary" to the Cedillos' claims. Id. at *1. Regarding some 23 expert witnesses who testified or submitted reports, he stated that "[t]he expert witnesses presented by the respondent were far better qualified, far more experienced, and far more persuasive than the petitioners' experts, concerning most of the key points." Id. While acknowledging that Michelle Cedillo "has tragically suffered from autism and other severe conditions," the Special Master concluded, "the petitioners have . . . failed to demonstrate that [Michelle's] vaccinations played any role at all in causing those problems." Id.

Petitioners timely filed their motion for review on March 16, 2009, raising seven arguments to support their position that the Special Master's decision is arbitrary, capricious, and not in accordance with law. Respondent filed a response memorandum on April 15, 2009, and the Court heard oral argument on July 7, 2009. Like the Special Master, the Court expresses its deep sympathy and admiration for the Cedillo family in caring for Michelle, and for the countless other families who deal with autism on a daily basis. However, for the reasons explained in detail below, the Court finds that Petitioners' arguments linking Michelle Cedillo's injuries to thimerosal and the MMR vaccine are without merit. Accordingly, the Court affirms the Special Master's February 12, 2009 decision.

Factual Background

Michelle Cedillo was born on August 30, 1994. Id. at *4. Mrs. Cedillo's pregnancy and Michelle's birth were uncomplicated. Id. Records from Michelle's visits to pediatricians during her first sixteen months indicate relatively normal health. Id. She experienced a few typical childhood ailments, such as an episode of vomiting and loose stools in March 1995, and constipation in June 1995. Id. At two months of age, she was able to fix her eyes and follow a moving object, and to become startled in response to a loud noise. Id. At one year, she spoke a few words, crawled on her knees, and pulled herself to stand. Id. She began walking at sixteen to eighteen months, although the record lacks precision on this point. See Transcript of Proceedings, 1332–33, June 11–26, 2007 ("Tr."); Ex. 28 at 207.

Michelle received two early hepatitis B vaccinations, one in the hospital shortly after her birth, and the second on September 27, 1994. Cedillo, at *4. She received a diphtheria/tetanus/pertussis ("DTP") vaccination on October 31, 1994, a hemophilus influenza vaccination on December 27, 1994, and a polio vaccination on March 8, 1995. Id. She also received a third hepatitis B vaccination on March 8, 1995. Id. She received a chicken-pox vaccination on September 6, 1995. Id. The DTP, hepatitis B, and hemophilus influenza vaccines all contained a small amount of thimerosal. Id.

On December 20, 1995, at fifteen months of age, Michelle received an MMR vaccination at the office of her pediatrician, Dr. Daniel Crawford, of Yuma Pediatrics. Id.; Ex. 8 at 2. She next visited her pediatrician on January 6, 1996. Cedillo, at *5. On that visit, Mrs. Cedillo reported to Dr. Crawford that, one week after the MMR vaccination, Michelle had developed a fever and rash. Id. Although the fever subsided, it spiked again on January 5, 1996 and was accompanied by a cough and "gagging to the point of vomiting." Id. On the morning of January 6, 1996, Michelle's temperature, taken at home, was 105.7 degrees. Id. Dr. Crawford later recorded her temperature as 100.3 degrees and noted that Michelle was crying and had a "purulent postnasal drip." Id. Dr. Crawford diagnosed her with "sinusitis vs. flu" and prescribed antibiotics. Id.

Michelle visited Yuma Pediatrics again on March 15, 1996 for her scheduled wellchild check-up at age eighteen months. Id.; Ex. 8 at 1. Her medical records from this visit do not reflect any significant problems, stating that she seemed to "hear well" and "stool[] well." Cedillo, at *5. However, Dr. Crawford noted that Michelle was "talking less since ill in [January]." Id. At this visit, Michelle received additional DTP and hemophilus influenza vaccinations, both of which contained thimerosal. Pet'r Br. 17. Michelle did not see a physician again for more than one year. Cedillo, at *5.

On April 24, 1997, Michelle visited another pediatrician, Dr. Emilia Matos, whose notes indicate that a "developmental delay [is] suspected" and that she was referring Michelle to a specialist for further evaluation. Id. On May 2, 1997, Dr. William Masland, a neurologist, noted in Michelle's medical history that at sixteen months, she had developed a fever of over 105 degrees two weeks after the MMR immunization and lasting four days. Id. He added, "[s]ince then she [had] lost her ability to verbalize" and concluded, "[i]t would appear that there was some neurological harm done at the time of the fevers. Whether this was a post-immunization phenomenon or a separate occurrence, would be very difficult to say." Id.

Following these doctors' visits in early 1997, medical records show that Michelle's development became quite abnormal. Id. On July 21, 1997, Dr. Karlsson Roth, a developmental psychologist, examined Michelle and diagnosed her with severe autism and profound mental retardation, concluding that her future potential would be "extremely limited." Id. Michelle's evaluations in later years confirmed these diagnoses. For example, on March 1, 1999, Dr. Ira Lott, a pediatric neurologist, determined that Michelle had "autism of a severe degree" and that she "[did] not have much in the way of communicative speech." Id.

In addition to her severe autism and mental retardation, Michelle has suffered significant gastrointestinal problems. Id. at *6. Medical records indicate that Michelle began experiencing chronic diarrhea in May 1999. Id. She also suffered symptoms in 2000 suggesting gastroesophageal reflux disease, erosive esophagitis, and fecal impaction. Id. Beginning in June 2000, Michelle underwent multiple upper and lower endoscopies. Id. at *6, 116.2 During one such procedure in January 2002, a tissue sample was taken from Michelle's intestine. Id. at *6. The Unigenetics Laboratory in Dublin, Ireland performed a "Measles Virus Detection" test on this tissue sample, and concluded in a March 15, 2002 report that "measles virus was detected" in the tissue. Id. However, as will be addressed below, Special Master Hastings determined that the Unigenetics test results were unreliable. Id. at *30, 46, 58–59.

Michelle also has experienced arthritis, uveitis (inflammation of the eyes), pancreatitis, and severe feeding problems, requiring the use of a feeding tube. Id. at *6, 122. In more recent years, she has suffered from a severe seizure disorder, resulting once in a fractured leg when she fell. Id. at *6. The Special Master rightly observed that Michelle Cedillo continually has "suffered from a tragic series of medical misfortunes." Id.

History of Proceedings

Petitioners Theresa and Michael Cedillo filed their claim for compensation under the Vaccine Act on December 9, 1998. Id. at *13. Initially, the Cedillos asserted that Michelle's MMR vaccine caused her to suffer an encephalopathy, which is a "Table Injury" under the Vaccine Act. Id.; Resp't Br. 2, Apr. 15, 2009. For a "Table Injury," the claimant must show that he or she received a vaccination listed on the Vaccine Injury Table, and suffered a listed injury within a prescribed period. Upon such a showing, the vaccine is presumed to have caused the injury, entitling the petitioner to compensation unless the respondent shows that the injury was caused by some other factor. 42 U.S.C. § 300aa-14; Pafford v. Sec'y of HHS, 451 F.3d 1352, 1355 (Fed. Cir. 2006) (citation omitted).

On January 14, 2002, the Cedillos changed their petition from a "Table Injury" claim to a "causation-in-fact" claim. Cedillo, at *13. Under the amended petition, the Cedillos alleged that vaccines containing thimerosal, in combination with the MMR vaccine, cause autism. Id. at *15. A "causation-in-fact" claim does not carry a presumption of causation, and places the burden on the petitioner to prove that the vaccination actually caused the injury in question. Capizzano v. Sec'y of HHS, 440 F.3d 1317, 1320 (Fed. Cir. 2006) (citations omitted).

Michelle Cedillo's case is one of approximately 5,000 Vaccine Act cases pending in this Court alleging that a child's autism or similar disorder was caused by one or more vaccines. Cedillo, at *7. The term "autism" describes a set of developmental disorders characterized by impairments in social interaction, impairments in verbal and non-verbal communication, and restricted or repetitive patterns of behavior. Id. On July 3, 2002, in an effort to manage this large group of autism cases, the Chief Special Master instituted an Omnibus Autism Proceeding ("OAP"). Id. at *8. Under the OAP procedures, a group of counsel known as the Petitioners' Steering Committee ("PSC"), selected from the attorneys representing petitioners in the autism cases, had the responsibility for developing and presenting evidence on the general causation issue of whether the vaccines in question could cause autism. Id. The Special Masters then would apply the PSC's evidence to individual cases. Id.

The Chief Special Master initially designated Special Master Hastings to preside over the OAP, and to resolve individual petitions alleging that vaccines or thimerosal cause autism. Id. at *9. On January 11, 2007, the Chief Special Master named two additional Special Masters, Denise Vowell and Patricia Campbell-Smith, to preside jointly with Special Master Hastings over the OAP. Id. The individual petitions were divided among these three Special Masters. Id. A petitioner could elect to opt out of the OAP at any time if he or she did not want to await the outcome of the general causation proceedings. Id. at *9 n.14.

From 2002 to 2006, the PSC engaged in discovery on the general causation issue. Id. at *9. On December 20, 2006 and again on January 9, 2007, the PSC proposed that the general causation evidence be divided among three separate theories: (1) the combination of the MMR vaccine and thimerosal-containing vaccines can cause autism; (2) thimerosal containing vaccines alone can cause autism; and (3) the MMR vaccine alone can cause autism. Id. The PSC proposed using Michelle Cedillo as a test case in June 2007 to present the first general causation theory. Id. The three Special Masters agreed to the PSC's proposal but directed the PSC to select two additional test cases falling within the same general causation theory. Id. at *10. Under this plan, the PSC would present its general causation evidence concerning the first theory, along with evidence specific to Michelle Cedillo's case, in June 2007, after which the PSC would present the specific evidence for the two additional test cases. Id. Thereafter, the Special Masters would use a similar approach for each of the other two general causation theories. Id.

The parties submitted a vast amount of evidence in the Cedillo case on the general causation theory that the MMR vaccine and thimerosal-containing vaccines can combine to cause autism. Id. Special Master Hastings conducted an evidentiary hearing in the Cedillo case during June 11–26, 2007 to hear both general causation evidence and evidence specific to Michelle Cedillo's case. Id.; Tr. 1-2917. Petitioners presented testimony from six expert witnesses: H. Vasken Aposhian, Ph.D. (toxicology); Vera Byers, M.D., Ph.D. (immunology); Karin Hepner, Ph.D. (molecular biology); Ronald Kennedy, Ph.D. (virology); Marcel Kinsbourne, M.D. (neurology); and Arthur Krigsman, M.D. (gastroenterology). Tr. 3, 301, 578A, 861, 1026. Petitioners also called Theresa Cedillo, Michelle's mother, to testify as a fact witness. Id. at 3, 301, 2874. Respondent presented testimony from nine expert witnesses: Jeffrey Brent, M.D., Ph.D. (toxicology); Stephen Bustin, Ph.D. (molecular biology); Edwin Cook, M.D. (psychiatry, genetics); Eric Fombonne, M.D., FRCPsych (pediatric psychiatry, epidemiology); Diane Griffin, M.D., Ph.D. (virology); Stephen Hanauer, M.D. (gastroenterology); Christine McCusker, M.D. M.Sc., FRCP (pediatric immunology); Brian Ward, M.D., M.Sc. (virology); and Max Wiznitzer, M.D. (pediatric neurology). Id. at 1216, 1560, 1793, 2074, 2280, 2498. Respondent also submitted expert reports from Robert Fujinami, Ph.D. (immunology), Michael Gershon, M.D. (neurogastroenterology), and Andrew Zimmerman, M.D. (pediatric neurology), but these experts did not testify. Resp't Br. 4. Nicholas Chadwick, Ph.D. testified as a fact witness for Respondent. Tr. 2280. Special Masters Vowell and Campbell-Smith heard all of the testimony in Cedillo so that they could apply the general causation evidence to the individual test cases assigned to them. Cedillo, at *10.

Special Master Campbell-Smith conducted an evidentiary hearing in Hazlehurst during October 15–18, 2007, and Special

Master Vowell conducted an evidentiary hearing in Snyder during November 5–9, 2007. Id. at *11. All three of the Special Masters attended these hearings. Id. In both Hazlehurst and Snyder, Special Master Hastings permitted the Cedillo Petitioners to submit additional general causation evidence, and Respondent to submit additional rebuttal evidence. Id. at *14. The parties filed extensive post-hearing briefs between November 2007 and February 2008, and Special Master Hastings closed the evidentiary record on July 30, 2008. Id. at *11, 14.

The evidentiary record in these cases easily is the largest of all cases presented to the Court in the history of the Vaccine Act. Michelle Cedillo's medical records alone comprise some 7,700 pages. Id. at *14. The parties filed 23 expert reports in Cedillo, and 50 expert reports in Hazlehurst and Snyder combined. Id. Fifteen expert witnesses testified in Cedillo, four in Hazlehurst, and eight in Snyder. Id. The hearing transcripts consist of 2,917 pages in Cedillo, 1,049 pages in Snyder, and 570 pages in Hazlehurst. Id. The record in the three cases also contains 939 medical journal articles, textbook excerpts, and other medical literature. Id. These materials, perhaps daunting even to medical professionals, relate to the subjects of neurology, gastroenterology, virology, immunology, molecular biology, toxicology, genetics, and epidemiology. Id. at *15.

On February 12, 2009, Special Master Hastings issued his decision denying the Cedillos' claim under the Vaccine Act. According to the Special Master, Petitioners failed to demonstrate that: (1) thimerosal-containing vaccines can harm infant immune systems in general, or that Michelle Cedillo's own thimerosal-containing vaccinations harmed her immune system; (2) the MMR vaccine can cause autism in general, or that Michelle Cedillo's own MMR vaccination contributed to her autism; (3) the MMR vaccine can cause gastrointestinal dysfunction in general, or that Michelle Cedillo's own MMR vaccination contributed to her gastrointestinal problems; or (4) Michelle Cedillo's own MMR vaccination caused her mental retardation or seizure disorder. Id. Furthermore, the Special Master deemed unreliable the testing Petitioners offered to show the presence of the measles virus in Michelle Cedillo and other autistic children. Id. The Special Master also found that the evidence concerning the causation of regressive autism combined with gastrointestinal dysfunction in some individuals did not persuasively show either or both conditions to be vaccine-related. Id.

On March 13, 2009, Petitioners filed a motion for reconsideration, requesting the Special Master to overturn his February 12,

2009 decision based on new evidence not available at the June 2007 hearing. Special Master Hastings denied the motion on March 16, 2009 because it was not filed within the 21-day period required by RCFC, Appendix B, Vaccine Rule 10(e). Cedillo v. Sec'y of HHS, No. 98-916V, 2009 WL 996299, at *1 (Fed. Cl. Spec. Mstr. Mar. 16, 2009). Even if Petitioners had timely filed their motion, the Special Master concluded that it would not be "in the interest of justice" to withdraw his decision. Id. On that same day, Petitioners filed with the Court their motion for review of the Special Master's decision.

References

American Psychiatric Association. 2000. *Diagnostic and Statistical Manual of Mental Disorders, Fourth Edition, Text Revision.* Washington, D.C.: American Psychiatric Association.

Autism and Developmental Disabilities Monitoring Network Surveillance Year 2002 Principal Investigators. 2007. "Prevalence of Autism Spectrum Disorders—Autism and Developmental Disabilities Monitoring Network, Fourteen Sites, United States, 2002." *Morbidity and Mortality Weekly Report, Surveillance Summaries* 56 (SS01): 12–28.

Autism and Developmental Disabilities Monitoring Network Surveillance Year 2000 Principal Investigators. 2007. "Prevalence of Autism Spectrum Disorders—Autism and Developmental Disabilities Monitoring Network, Six Sites, United States, 2000." *Morbidity and Mortality Weekly Report, Surveillance Summaries* 56 (SS01): 1–11.

Barnea-Goraly, N., H. Kwon, V. Menon, L. Lotspeich, and A. Reiss. 2004. "White Matter Structure in Autism: Preliminary Evidence from Diffusion Tensor Imaging." *Biological Psychiatry* 55 (3): 323–26.

Baron-Cohen, S., H. Ring, E. Bullmore, S. Wheelwright, C. Ashwin, and S. Williams. 2000. "The Amygdala Theory of Autism." *Neuroscience and Biobehavioral Reviews* 24 (3): 355–64.

Bauman, M., and T. Kemper. 2005. "Neuroanatomic Observations of the Brain in Autism: A Review and Future Directions." *International Journal of Developmental Neuroscience* 23 (2–3): 183–87.

Bentin, S., T. Allison, A. Puce, E. Perez, and G. McCarthy. 1996. "Electrophysiological Studies of Face Perception in Humans." *Journal of Cognitive Neuroscience* 8 (6): 551–65.

Brothers, L. 1990. "The Social Brain: A Project for Integrating Primate Behavior and Neurophysiology in a New Domain." *Concepts in Neuroscience* 1:27–51.

Bushnell, I., F. Sai, and J. Mullin. 1989. "Neonatal Recognition of the Mother's Face." *British Journal of Developmental Pscyhology* 7:3–15.

Charman, T., and P. Clare. 2004. *Mapping Autism Research: Identifying UK Priorities for the Future.* London: National Autistic Society.

Cohen, M., and D. Eisenberg. 2002. "Potential Physician Malpractice Liability Associated with Complementary and Integrative Medical Therapies." *Annals of Internal Medicine* 136:596–603.

Courchesne, E. 1997. "Brainstem, Cerebellar and Limbic Neuro-anatomical Abnormalities in Autism." *Current Opinions in Neurobiology* 7 (2): 269–78.

Croen, L., D. Najjar, G. Ray, L. Lotspeich, and Bernal, P. 2006. "A Comparison of Health Care Utilization and Costs of Children with and without Autism Spectrum Disorders in a Large Group-Model Health Plan." *Pediatrics* 118:e1203–e1211.

Dapretto, M., M. Davies, J. Pfeifer, A. Scott, M. Sigman, S., Bookheimer, and M. Iacoboni. 2006. "Understanding Emotions in Others: Mirror Neuron Dysfunction in Children with Autism Spectrum Disorders." *Nature Neuroscience* 9 (1): 28–30.

Dawson, G., S. J. Webb, and J. McPartland. 2005. "Understanding the Nature of Face Processing Impairment in Autism: Insights from Behavioral and Electrophysiological Studies. *Developmental Neuropsychology* 27 (3): 403–24.

Dawson, G., and K. Zanolli. 2003. "Early Intervention and Brain Plasticity in Autism." *Novartis Foundation Symposium* 251: 266–74; discussion 274–80, 281–97

Dawson, G., A. Meltzoff, J. Osterling, and J, Rinaldi. 1998. "Neuropsychological Correlates of Early Symptoms of Autism." *Child Development* 69 (5): 1276–85.

de Haan, M., M. Johnson, and H. Halit. 2003. "Development of Face-sensitive Event-related Potentials during Infancy: A Review." *International Journal of Psychophysiology* 51:45–58.

Dyches, T., L. Wilder, and F. Obiakor. 2001. "Autism: Multicultural Perspectives." In *Autistic Spectrum Disorders: Educational and Clinical Interventions,* ed. T. Wahlberg, F. Obiakor, S. Burkhardt, and A. F. Rotatori, 151–77. Oxford: Elsevier Science.

Exhorn, K. S. 2005. *The Autism Sourcebook.* New York: Regan.

Farah, M. J., J. Tanaka, and H. Drain. 1995. "What Causes the Face Inversion Effect?" *Journal of Experimental Psychology and Human Perceptual Performance* 21:628–34.

Filipek, P., P. Accardo, S. Ashwal, G. Baranek, E. Cook, G. Dawson, B. Gordon, et al. 2000. "Practice Parameter: Screening and Diagnosis of Autism: Report of the Quality Standards Subcommittee of the American Academy of Neurology and the Child Neurology Society." *Neurology* 55 (4): 468–79.

Freeman, B. J. 1997. "Guidelines for Evaluating Intervention Programs for Children with Autism." *Journal of Autism and Developmental Disorders* 27:641–51.

Ganz, M. 2009. "The Lifetime Distribution of the Incremental Societal Costs of Autism." *Archives of Pediatric and Adolescent Medicine* 161: 343–49.

Ganz, M. L. 2006. "The Costs of Autism." In *Understanding Autism: From Basic Neuroscience to Treatment,* ed. S. O. Moldin and J. L. R. Rubenstein, 475–502. Boca Raton, FL: Taylor and Francis Group.

Goren, C., M. Sarty, and P. Wu. 1975. "Visual Following and Pattern Discrimination of Face-like Stimuli by Newborn Infants. *Pediatrics* 56:544–49.

Guevara, J., D. Mandell, A. Rostain, H. Zhao, and T. Hadley. 2003. "National Estimates of Health Services Expenditures for Children with Behavioral Disorders: An Analysis of the Medical Expenditure Panel Survey." *Pediatrics* 112 (6): e440.

Gurney, J., M. Fritz, K. Ness, P. Sievers, C. Newschaffer, and E. Shapiro. 2003. "Analysis of Prevalence Trends of Autism Spectrum Disorder in Minnesota." *Archives of Pediatric and Adolescent Medicine* 157 (7): 622–27.

Haxby, J., B. Horwitz, L. Ungerleider, J. Maisog, P. Pietrini, and C. Grady. 1994. "The Functional Organization of Human Extrastriate Cortex: A Pet-rCBF Study of Selective Attention to Faces and Locations." *The Journal of Neuroscience* 14:6336–53.

Hobson, R. 1986. "The Autistic Child's Appraisal of Expressions of Emotion." *Journal of Child Psychology and Psychiatry* 27 (3): 321–42.

Howlin, P., I. Magiati, and T. Charman. 2009. "Systematic Review of Early Intensive Behavioral Interventions for Children with Autism." *American Journal of Intellectual Development and Disabilities* 114 (1): 23.

Johnson, M. H., S. Dziurawiec, H. Ellis, and J. Morton. 1991. "Newborns' Preferential Tracking of Face-like Stimuli and Its Subsequent Decline." *Cognition* 40 (1–2): 1–19.

Kanwisher, N., J. McDermott, and M. M. Chun. 1997. "The Fusiform Face Area: A Module in Human Extrastriate Cortex Specialized for Face Perception." *Journal of Neuroscience* 17 (11): 4302–11.

Kleinhans, N., T. Richards, L. Sterling, K. Stegbauer, R. Mahurin, L. Johnson, J. Greenson, G. Dawson, and E. Aylward. 2008. "Abnormal Functional Connectivity in Autism Spectrum Disorders during Face Processing." *Brain* 131 (4): 1000–1012.

Klin, A., W. Jones, R. Schultz, F. Volkmar, and D. Cohen. 2002. "Visual Fixation Patterns during Viewing of Naturalistic Social Situations as Predictors of Social Competence in Individuals with Autism." *Archives of General Psychiatry* 59 (9): 809–16.

Kogan, M., S. Blumberg, L. Schieve, C. Boyle, J. Perrin, R. Ghandour, G. Singh, B. Strickland, E. Trevathan, and P. van Dyck. 2009. "Prevalence of Parent-Reported Diagnosis of Autism Spectrum Disorder among Children in the US, 2007." *Pediatrics* 124:.

Leppanen, J., and C. Nelson. 2009. "Tuning the Developing Brain to Social Signals of Emotions." *Nature Reviews: Neuroscience* 10:37–47.

Lovaas, O. 1987. "Behavioral Treatment and Normal Educational and Intellectual Functioning in Young Autistic Children." *Journal of Consulting and Clinical Psychology* 55 (1): 3–9.

Mandell, D., R. Ittenbach, S. Levy, and J. Pinto-Martin. 2007. "Disparities in Diagnoses Received Prior to a Diagnosis of Autism Spectrum Disorder." *Journal of Autism and Developmental Disorders* 37 (9): 1795–802.

Mandell, D., J. Listerud, S. Levy, and J. Pinto-Martin. 2002. "Race Differences in the Age at Diagnosis among Medicaid-eligible Children with Autism." *Journal of American Academy of Child and Adolescent Psychiatry* 41 (12): 1447–53.

McPartland, J., Dawson, G., Webb, S., Panagiotides, H., and Carver, L. 2004. "Event-related Brain Potentials Reveal Anomalies in Temporal Processing of Faces in Autism Spectrum Disorder." *Journal of Child Psychology and Psychiatry* 45 (7): 1235–45.

Meltzoff, A. N., and M. K. Moore. 1977. "Imitation of Facial and Manual Gestures by Human Neonates." *Science* 198 (4312): 74–78.

Minshew, N. J., and D. L. Williams. 2007. "The New Neurobiology of Autism: Cortex, Connectivity, and Neuronal Organization." *Archives of Neurology* 64 (7): 945–50.

Mundy, P. 2003. "Annotation: The Neural Basis of Social Impairments in Autism: The Role of the Dorsal Medial-Frontal Cortex and Anterior Cingulate System." *Journal of Child Psychology and Psychiatry* 44 (6): 793–80.

Murias, M., Webb, S., Greenson, J., and Dawson, G. 2007. "Resting State Cortical Connectivity Reflected in EEG Coherence in Individuals with Autism." *Biological Psychiatry* 62 (3): 270–73.

Myers, S. M., C. P. Johnson, and American Academy of Pediatrics Council on Children With Disabilities. 2007. "Management of Children with Autism Spectrum Disorders." *Pediatrics* 120 (5): 1162–82.

Newacheck, P., and S. Kim. 2005. "A National Profile of Health Care Utilization and Expenditures for Children with Special Health Care Needs." *Archives of Pediatric and Adolescent Medicine* 159:10–17.

Newschafer, C., M. Falb, and J. Gurney. 2005. "National Autism Prevalence Trends from United States Special Education Data." *Pediatrics* 115:277–82.

Osterling, J., and G. Dawson. 1994. "Early Recognition of Children with Autism: A Study of First Birthday Home Videotapes." *Journal of Autism & Developmental Disorders* 24 (3): 247–57.

Pelphrey, K., and E. Carter. 2008. "Charting the Typical and Atypical Development of the Social Brain." *Developmental Psychopathology* 20 (4): 1081–102

Puce, A., T. Allison, J. Gore, and G. McCarthy. 1995. "Face-sensitive Regions in Human Extrastriate Cortex Studied by Functional MRI." *Journal of Neurophysiology,* 74 (3): 1192–99.

Schultz, R. T., I. Gauthier, A. Klin, R. Fulbright, A. Anderson, F. Volkmar, P. Skudlarski, C. Lacadie, D. Cohen, and J. Gore. 2000. "Abnormal Ventral Temporal Cortical Activity during Face Discrimination among Individuals with Autism and Asperger Syndrome." *Archives of General Psychiatry* 57 (4): 331–40.

7

Directory of Organizations

Private, Not-for-Profit Organizations

Association for Retarded Citizens (ARC)

Web site: http://www.thearc.org/NetCommunity/Page.
aspx?pid=183

The ARC advocates for individuals with intellectual and developmental disabilities to ensure full participation in the community. By working with members, the ARC strives to provide support for the active engagement and success of individuals with intellectual disability. Since its establishment in 1950 by parents, when little was known about mental retardation, the ARC has worked to educate the public regarding mental retardation and help to obtain services for those impacted by mental retardation and developmental disabilities.

Association for Science in Autism Treatment (ASAT)

Web site: http://asatonline.org/

The mission of ASAT is to provide accurate, scientifically based information regarding autism and intervention. There is so much information available about autism but the quality of information that is available varies considerably. There is a great deal of misinformation regarding the causes of autism and the effectiveness of treatments. ASAT strives to provide clear, accurate, and scientific understanding regarding autism to families and individuals and reduce the misinformation about the disorder.

Autism and PDD Support Network

Web site: http://www.autism-pdd.net/

The Autism and PDD support network is an online community and resource center for families affected by autism spectrum disorders. Through the community's Web site, viewers can review resources and information, review forum postings and post questions and share concerns.

Autism National Committee (AUTCOM)

Web site: http://www.autcom.org/

AUTCOM is an advocacy organization committed to support "Social Justice for All Citizens with Autism." Founded in 1990 to protect the human rights of individuals with an autism spectrum disorder, AUTCOM currently hosts a Web site with information regarding political discourse, judicial decisions, advocacy issues, educational information, book reviews, and a newsletter.

Autism Research Institute (ARI)

Web site: http://www.autism.com/

The ARI was founded in 1967 by Dr. Bernard Rimland, an experimental psychologist, parent of a child with autism, and one of the founders of the Autism Society of America. Dr. Rimland was a strong advocate for the biological basis of autism during a time when psychoanalytic theories held sway (see Chapter 2 for a historical perspective). The ARI is committed to fostering research to improve diagnosis, treatment and prevention of autism. The ARI maintains a large databank of case histories and publishes a quarterly newsletter. Additionally, in 1995, the ARI established and continues to support Defeat Autism Now! (DAN!), a project focused on the education of parents and professionals regarding biomedical treatments for autism. The ARI also sponsors Autism Television (http://www.up-to-date.com/autism.tv/index.html), which provides a number of video and audio channels showcasing organizations and events such as the ARI and DAN! conferences.

Autism Science Foundation (ASF)

Web site: http://autismsciencefoundation.org

The ASF was founded in 2009 by Alison Singer, formerly of Autism Speaks, and Karen London, one of the founding members of National Alliance for Autism Research, to fund research based on rigorous scientific standards and values. The ASF bases its mission on the principles that autism has a strong genetic component and research should focus on the mechanisms that trigger autism; that research into evidence-based, effective lifespan interventions is needed; and that "vaccines save lives; they do not cause autism" and research dollars into a vaccine autism link is not warranted.

Autism Society of America

Web site: http://www.autism-society.org

The Autism Society of America was founded in 1965 by Dr. Bernard Rimland, Dr. Ruth Sullivan, and a group of parents of children with autism as a grassroots advocacy organization. The mission of the organization is improve the lives of all individuals with autism by increasing public awareness, advocating for the provision of services, and disseminating information about treatment, research, and education. With a strong chapter network and a national board of directors that includes individuals with autism, a panel of professional advisors, and a panel of "people on the spectrum of autism" advisors, the organization hosts a large national conference, publishes a quarterly newsletter, and maintains a large Web presence. Additionally, the organization maintains a large information and referral database and service and a Web site that is in both English and Spanish.

Autism Speaks

Web site: http://www.autismspeaks.org

Autism Speaks is a not for profit organization focused on raising public awareness of autism, funding and supporting research into the "causes, prevention, treatments, and cure" for autism, with a defined goal to "change the future for all who struggled with autism spectrum disorders." Bob and Suzanne Wright founded Autism Speaks in 2005 after their grandson was diagnosed with autism. In its first year it raised $40 million to fund autism research and was able to establish a number of research programs and support independent research projects.

During its first years, Autism Speaks made a number of mergers with other nonprofit organizations. In 2005 Autism Speaks merged with Autism Coalition for Research and Education (ACRE). ACRE was an organization founded by parents in 1998 to support biomedical and applied research and increase public awareness. In January of 2006, Autism Speaks merged with the National Alliance for Autism Research (NAAR). NAAR was the first nonprofit, founded in 1994, dedicated to supporting research in the causes and treatments for autism. During a time when limited funds were available through federal programs for autism research, Karen and Eric London, parents of a child with autism, joined forces with professionals to raise money and accelerate the pace of autism research. Prior to the merger with Autism Speaks, NAAR committed more than $20 million to research through collaborative projects, fellowships, and research programs. NAAR established the Autism Tissue Program, a brain tissue program that Autism Speaks continues to maintain. A third merger in 2007, included Cure Autism Now (CAN). Jonathan Shestack and Portia Iversen, parents of a child with autism, founded CAN in 1995 to support research in the prevention, treatment and cure of autism. CAN, through the provision of close to $40 million dollars to autism research, developed and supported a number of programs that Autism Speaks maintains including the Autism Genetics Research Exchange, a genetics repository, and the Clinical Trials Network, a program focused on translating basic science to clinical applications.

In 2009 Alison Singer, the vice president of communications and awareness for Autism Speaks resigned citing a difference of opinion regarding Autism Speaks' policy on immunization research. Given the limited research funding available, Alison Singer reported a need to focus on other avenues of research. She, along with Eric London, one of the founding members of NAAR who also resigned from the Autism Speaks board, shortly thereafter founded the Autism Science Foundation.

AutismSpot

Web site: http://www.autismspot.com/about

AutismSpot.com's mission is "empowering the autism community" through the provision of information and resources through an organization that is not supported by donations or government funding. The founders aim to remain unbiased in the information that is provided via the multimedia Web site.

Consortium for Citizens with Disabilities (CCD)

Web site: http://www.c-c-d.org

CCD is national advocacy coalition of consumer, advocacy, provider and professional organizations working in the field of disabilities. The aim of the coalition is to fully integrate children and adults with disabilities into mainstream society.

Council for Learning Disabilities (CLD)

Web site: http://www.cldinternational.org

CLD is an international organization with a mission to improve the quality of life for individuals with learning disabilities and challenges in learning. Made up of professionals, the organization promotes evidence-based methods of instruction as well as research into learning disabilities and advocacy for individuals with learning disabilities. The CLD has a number of regional chapters throughout the United States, supports two professional publications, hosts conferences, and provides information for professionals.

Doug Flutie Jr. Foundation for Autism

Web site: http://www.dougflutiejrfoundation.org

The Doug Flutie Jr. Foundation for Autism was founded in 2000 by the NFL quarterback Doug Flutie Sr. and his wife, Laurie. As parents of a child with autism, they wanted to provide families of children with autism with resources and support. The foundation supports nonprofit organizations that provide clinical services to children with autism and organizations that conduct research on the causes and effects of autism.

Families for Early Autism Treatment (FEAT)

Web site: http://www.feat.org/

FEAT is a nonprofit organization focused on providing advocacy, education and support around autism spectrum disorders. FEAT maintains a Web site, newsletter, email list, and resource information. Originally started in 1993 in northern California, FEAT has grown to include 24 U.S. chapters and 3 Canadian chapters with a specific focus on empirically supported interventions.

Families of Adults Afflicted with Asperger's Syndrome (FAAAS)

Web site: http://faaas.org

The mission of the nonprofit FAAAS is to support family members of adult individuals with Asperger's Disorder. The focus of the organization is to generate public awareness about Asperger's Disorder in the adult population, provide support for family members, and disseminate education through the Web site, mailing list, and conferences.

First Signs

Web site: http://www.firstsigns.org/

First Signs mission is to provide education about the early warning signs of autism spectrum disorders. By improving screening practices and lowering the age at which children are diagnosed with developmental disorders the organization aims to improve outcomes for children with disabilities. First Signs maintains a comprehensive Web site with resources, news updates, a video glossary, and opportunity for sharing.

Foundation for Educating Children with Autism (FECA)

Web site: http://www.fecainc.org
Contact: questions@FEACinc.org

FECA is a national nonprofit with a focus on providing educational opportunities based on applied behavioral analysis principles to children with autism. FECA was founded in 1994 by eight families concerned about the educational opportunities available for their children with autism. Through the establishment of schools, training of professionals, community outreach, and advocacy, the organization aims to improve the lives of individuals with autism.

Generation Rescue

Web site: http://www.generationrescue.org/index.html

Generation Rescue is a parent-founded and parent-led nonprofit focused on biomedical treatments for autism. Jenny McCarthy and Jim Carrey play a prominent role in Generation Rescue as members of the board of directors. Generation Rescue is part of the Autism Collaboration, a collection of advocacy organizations that includes NAA, SafeMinds, ASA, ARI, and others.

The Help Group

Web site: http://www.thehelpgroup.org

The Help Group is a comprehensive nonprofit organization that serves children with special needs including autism spectrum disorders. The Help Group runs seven specialized day schools in the Los Angeles area, but provides public awareness, professional training, and parent education programs at both the state and national level.

Interactive Autism Network (IAN)

Web site: http://www.iancommunity.org/

IAN is an online community of Kennedy Krieger Institute and sponsored by Autism Speaks with a goal to facilitate research in understanding and treating autism spectrum disorders. The IAN community Web site provides an online meeting place for researchers and families alike where information regarding the latest research can be presented and discussed.

MAAP Services for Autism and Asperger Syndrome

Web site: http://maapservices.org/

Founded in 1984 by a parent of a daughter with autism, MAAP is a nonprofit with a mission to provide information and advice to "families of More advanced individuals with Autism, Asperger's syndrome, and Pervasive Developmental Disorder" (MAAP). MAAP provides a quarterly newsletter, a Web site, and state-by-state professional and parent support listing.

Manitas por Autismo (SPANISH)

Web site: http://www.manitasporautismo.com/

Manitas por Autismo is a parent-run, nonprofit organization focused on dissemination of autism information for Spanish speaking families. The vision of the organization is to develop a better standard of living for Latino families affected by autism. Through the organization's Web site information and news regarding autism, a directory of international organizations, and a community forum is provided.

Mothers United for Moral Support (MUMS)

Web site: http://www.netnet.net/mums/

MUMS is a parent-founded, national support organization with a main mission to provide support for parents of children with disabilities through a parent network system. Through the organization parents are matched with other parents whose children have the same disability or condition with considerations to age, geographical location, gender, and symptom severity included in the matching.

National Alliance on Mental Illness (NAMI)

Web site: http://www.nami.org

NAMI is a grassroots advocacy organization dedicated to increasing public awareness about mental illness. The organization also provides information via their Web site about current events, legislative action, and mental illness and developmental disorders, including autism spectrum disorders

National Autism Association (NAA)

Web site: http://nationalautismassociation.org

NAA is a parent-founded nonprofit with a mission to educate and empower families affected with autism and to advocate for individuals who are unable to advocate for themselves. As part of the mission statement the organization poses that autism is not a genetic disorder but "one that is biomedically definable and treatable" and propose that environmental toxins are causative factors in autism. NAA is part of the Autism Collaboration, a collection of advocacy organizations that includes NAA, SafeMinds, ASA, ARI, Generation Rescue, and others.

National Disability Rights Network (NDRN)

Web site: http://www.napas.org

The NDRN is a nonprofit membership organization that serves individuals with disability with an aim to create a society with equal opportunities and full participation of individuals with disabilities in society. The network includes disability rights organizations and through the Web site the organization provides information regarding disability rights.

National Rehabilitation Information Center (NARIC)

Web site: http://www.naric.com

NARIC collects and disseminates the research findings and results from the National Institutes on Disability and Rehabilitation

Research (NIDRR). NARIC also provides information to the disability and rehabilitation communities through a comprehensive Web site, a toll free referral service, an electronic bulletin board to improve access for libraries and research institutions, online directories, and a fully interactive online rehabilitation database.

Organization for Autism Research (OAR)

Web site: http://www.researchautism.org

Founded in 2001 by a group of parents and grandparents of children and adults with autism spectrum disorders, OAR aims to use applied science to address questions facing the autism community. OAR funds pilot studies and targeted research into the behavioral and social development of individuals with autism with a focus on communication, education, and vocational challenges. Additionally, on the comprehensive Web site, OAR provides information for educators, professionals and families regarding autism spectrum disorders including providing worksheets and planning tools for educational programs. Additionally, there is information for families concerning participation in research that includes basic information about scientific research, a parent's guide to research, and a searchable database for research institutions.

SafeMinds

Web site: http://safeminds.org/

SafeMinds is a nonprofit organization with a mission to support research, raise awareness, change policy and focus national attention on a proposed link between mercury and autism. The debate on a possible link between mercury and autism persists and is a significant controversy in the history of autism. SafeMinds is part of the Autism Collaboration, a collection of advocacy organizations that includes NAA, ASA, ARI, Generation Rescue, and others.

Sibling Support Project

Web site: http://siblingsupport.org/

The Sibling Support Project is a program of the Kindering Center with funding from the Wilson Foundation and is an effort to address the concerns of siblings of individuals with developmental disabilities, autism, or other mental health concerns. By training local providers in how to provide support programs for siblings, hosting workshops, disseminating information on the organization's Web site and Listserv, and increasing awareness of sibling concerns, the organization aims to accomplish this mission.

Simons Foundation Autism Research Initiative (SFARI)

Web site: http://sfari.org/

The Simons Foundation is a philanthropic foundation that focuses on supporting work in math, science, and autism. SFARI is the arm of the foundation focusing on autism research, specifically research to improve diagnosis, treatment and prevention of autism. In 2003, the Simons Foundation hosted a roundtable on autism research. At this meeting of top minds in epidemiology, neuroscience, psychiatry, and autism convened and through the productive discussion research initiatives were developed. SFARI funds a large number of projects from independent scientists focusing on understanding autism primarily from the perspective of cognitive neuroscience and genetics. A major initiative of the Simons Foundation is the Simons Simplex Collection (SSC)—an international collaboration of scientists focusing on exploring the genetics of autism.

Talk about Curing Autism (TACA)

Web site: http://www.talkaboutcuringautism.org

TACA is a nonprofit organization that provides information, resources, and support to families affected by autism. TACA was founded in 2000 by a group of parents based in California and in 2008 launched chapters in nine other states. With a number of education and support meetings sponsored by state chapters, the *TACA Autism Journey Guide*—a freely available resource book developed by TACA—a parent mentorship program, the Web site (in English and Spanish), loaner libraries, and family scholarships, the organization provides information and support for families just receiving a diagnosis of autism with an aim to speed the process from diagnosis to treatment. Information that is provided ranges from empirically supported behavioral treatments to biomedical and dietary interventions. TACA is part of the Autism Collaboration, a collection of advocacy organizations that includes NAA, ASA, ARI, Unlocking Autism, Generation Rescue, and others.

Unlocking Autism

Web site: http://www.unlockingautism.org

Unlocking Autism was founded in 1999 by parents and grandparents with a mission to gather information about how to help children with autism and disseminate that information quickly to parents of newly diagnosed children. Through parent education about biomedical and behavioral interventions, pending legislation, and laws; funding for biomedical and behavioral research and projects; and a nationwide parent to parent hotline for parents of newly diagnosed children the organization aims to "bring the issues of autism form individual homes to the forefront of national dialogue." Unlocking autism is part of the Autism Collaboration, a collection of advocacy organizations that includes NAA, ASA, ARI, Generation Rescue, TACA, and others.

Professional Organizations

American Academy of Pediatricians (AAP)

Web site: http://www.aap.org

The AAP is a professional organization consisting of approximately 60,000 physicians with a specialty in pediatric medicine throughout several countries. By supporting the professional needs of its constituents the organization aims to "attain optimal physical, mental and social health and well being for all infants, children, adolescents, and young adults." The AAP publishes a number of position papers including manuscripts focused on the identification and treatment of autism. Additionally, on the organization's Web site information, links, and resources focusing on autism is provided on the "Children's Health Topics" Web page.

American Speech and Hearing Association (ASHA)

Web site: http://www.asha.org

ASHA is the national, professional, scientific, and credentialing organization for speech-language pathologists, audiologists, and speech, language, and hearing scientists. With a mission to advocate for individuals with communication and related disorders, to advance communication science, and promote effective human communication, the organization provides information for professionals and the public regarding communication and related disorders, including autism spectrum disorders.

Council for Exceptional Children (CEC)

Web site: http://www.cec.sped.org

The CEC is a professional organization focused on improving educational success of individuals with disabilities and/or exceptional talents. The CEC lobbies for appropriate governmental policies, sets professional standards, advocates for individuals with exceptional abilities, and provides professional development opportunities.

Governmental Organizations

Autism Coordinating Center

Web site: http://www.nichd.nih.gov/autism/research.cfm

In 1997, under direction from Congress, the Autism Coordinating Center was established by the National Institutes of Health to improve the quality, speed and coordination of efforts at NIH in finding a cure for autism. The Autism Coordinating Center is comprised of NIH institutes: Eunice Kennedy Shriver National Institutes of Child Health and Human Development (NICHD); National Institutes on Deafness and Other Communication Disorders (NIDCD); National Institutes for Mental Health (NIMH); National Institutes of Neurological Disorders and Stroke (NINDS); National Institutes of Environmental Health Sciences (NIEHS). Other organizations and representatives participate in Autism

Coordinating Center meetings for specific topics. The Autism Coordinating Center is cochaired by the directors of NIMH and NICHD.

Centers for Disease Control and Prevention (CDC)

Main Web site: http://www.cdc.gov
Autism Spectrum Disorders site: http://www.cdc.gov/ncbddd/autism/index.html
Learn the Signs. Act Early page: http://www.cdc.gov/ncbddd/actearly/index.html

The CDC is a major component of the U.S. Department of Health and Human Services with a mission to provide the expertise and tools so that people and communities can protect their health. The CDC sponsors and coordinates research into autism spectrum disorders and provides information for professionals and the public regarding autism, developmental screening and early warning signs, and resources and links for services and programs through the comprehensive Web site.

Clinical Trials.gov

Web site: http://www.clinicaltrials.gov/

ClinicalTrials.gov is a service of the National Institutes of Health coordinated by the National Library of Medicine. ClinicalTrials.gov is a registry of clinical trials being conducted in the United States and internationally that are both federally and privately funded. Through the organization's Web site, readers can learn about the purpose of the clinical trials, the eligibility requirements for participation in studies, the location of the studies, and contact information for each trial.

Interagency Autism Coordinating Committee (IACC)

Web site: http://iacc.hhs.gov/

The IACC coordinates all the activities related to ASDs that are supported by the Department of Health and Human Services. The IACC was established in accordance with the Combating Autism Act of 2006. The IACC membership is comprised of both federal and public members. The director of the National Institutes for Mental Health chairs the committee. There are twelve federal committee members, including the director of the National Institutes on Deafness and Other Communication Disorders, the director of the National Institutes of Health, the director of the National Center on Birth Defects and Developmental Disabilities from the Centers for Disease Control and Prevention, the director of the National Institutes of Environmental Health Sciences, the director of the Office on Disability, and seven others. There are six public committee members on the IACC including the president and CEO of the Autism Society of America, the president of the Autism Science Foundation, and four others. There is an additional subcommittee focused on assessing and improving services and supports for people with ASD. Each full and subcommittee meeting of the IACC is open to the public and the committee requests public comment during each meeting. The committee prepared a summary of advances in autism research during the calendar year in 2008, which is available, along with strategic plan reports and other IACC publications on the IACC Web site.

National Dissemination Center for Children with Disabilities

Web site: http://www.nichcy.org

The National Dissemination Center for Children with Disabilities is a service center funding by the Office of Special Education Programs, in the U.S. Department of Education and is operated by the Academy for Educational Development. The center provides information regarding disabilities in children, programs and services for children with disabilities, and information about special education laws. The center maintains a toll free hotline (1-800-695-0285) for both English and Spanish speakers, a monthly newsletter, an eNews service for which children or families can register to receive news bulletin specific to their indicated topics of, and a bilingual Web site. On the Web site, information regarding specific disabilities (including autism), early intervention, special education, individualized education programs (IEPs), education rights and laws, research on education and intervention, disability organizations, and the transition process to adulthood for individuals with disabilities, is available. Additionally, on the Web site there is state specific information regarding organizations, associations, and agencies that address disability issues.

National Institutes for Health Autism Research Networks

Web site: http://www.autismresearchnetwork.org/AN/default.aspx
—Collaborative Programs of Excellence in Autism (CPEA)
—Studies to Advance Autism Research and Treatment Network (STAART)
—Autism Centers of Excellence (ACE)

The CPEA was started in 1997 by the National Institutes of Child Health and Human Development (NICHD) in collaboration with the National Institutes on Deafness and Other Communication Disorders (NIDCD) as a five-year, $45 million, international network to explore the neurobiology and genetics of autism. Funding was renewed for an additional five years. The network included 10 sites linking 129 scientists from the United States and seven other countries and involved more than 2,000 families with autism in a number of projects focused on identifying the genetic, immunological, and environmental risk factors for autism. The CPEA centers were Boston University, University of California–Davis, University of California–Los Angeles, University of Pittsburgh, University of Rochester Medical Center, University of Texas Health Science Center at Houston, University of Utah, University of Washington, and Yale University.

The STAART network was established in response to the Children's Health Act of 2000. The Act called for the establishment of five centers of excellence in autism research, but the five NIH Institutes involved in the NIH Autism Coordinating Committee [Eunice Kennedy Shriver NICHD; NIDCD; National Institutes for Mental Health (NIMH); National Institutes of Neurological Disorders and Stroke (NINDS); National Institutes of Environmental Health Sciences (NIEHS)] funded eight centers to focus on the causes, diagnosis, early detection, prevention, and treatment of autism. Each center supported three or more projects, with at least one study focused on treatment. The eight STAART centers were Boston University, Kennedy Krieger Institute, Mount Sinai, University of California-Los Angeles, University of North Carolina, University of Rochester, University of Washington and Yale University.

In 2007 the National Institutes of Health implemented the ACE program, which is a consolidation of the CPEA and STAART programs. The ACE program includes both ACE centers, in which collaborations between specialists in a range of fields collaborate in autism research to answer a range of research questions, and ACE networks, in which scientists at research facilities across the country collaborate to address a single research question. All ACE program award recipients participate in the National Database for Autism Research (NDAR), which is a National Institutes of Health, Web-based database tool that allows researchers around the world to collect and share information on autism. In the first year of the program, five centers and two networks were awarded. The five centers include the University of Illinois–Chicago, the University of California–San Diego, the University of California–Los Angeles, the University of Pittsburgh, and the University of Washington. In the second year of the program, additional centers were established. The two network recipients were the University of North Carolina–Chapel Hill and the University of California–Davis. In 2008, the second year of the ACE program, an additional center, Yale University, was added. Three additional ACE networks were awarded to Wayne State University, University of California–Los Angeles, and Drexel University.

National Institutes for Mental Health (NIMH)

Web site: http://www.nimh.nih.gov

NIHM is an institute of the National Institutes of Health established in 1949 that generates research and promotes research training that focuses on the understanding, treatment and prevention of mental illness. The vision of the institute is that of a world in which mental illnesses are prevented and cured. The four objectives of the NIMH are to promote the discovery of the etiology of mental disorders; to understand when, where and how to intervene in mental illness; to develop new and more effective interventions for mental illness that take into account the diversity of individuals; and expand the public health impact of research into mental illness. The institute maintains a Web site with information on mental health and mental illness; science news in the field of mental health; information on research opportunities, studies, and events; and announcements from the NIMH. In addition to specific health information, free publications, statistics concerning mental health, links to other resources, and outreach information are available through the institute. The NIMH maintains a specific Web page focusing on autism, including information about the disorder, links to other resources, and current research on the disorder.

National Institutes of Child Health and Human Development (NICHD)

Web site: http://www.nichd.nih.gov

The NICHD is an institute of the National Institutes of Health established in 1962 that conducts and supports research that focuses on the health of children and families. Areas of focus include: infant death reduction, reproductive health, birth defects, mental retardation, developmental disabilities, growth and development, rehabilitation research, and the health of women, men and families. The organization maintains a Web site with information on health and human development topics, which includes health education, information about publications and other materials, and information regarding research conducted at NICHD and supported by the NICHD. The NICHD maintains a Web page focusing on autism, including information about the disorder, links to other resources, and freely downloadable informational publications.

National Institutes of Health (NIH)

Web site: http://www.nih.gov

The NIH is part of the U.S. Department of Health and Human Services and is the nation's medical research agency charged with conducting and supporting medical research. The roots of the NIH began in 1887 when a one-room laboratory was created in the Marine Hospital Service, which later became the U.S. Public Health Service. Since these early beginnings, the NIH has expanded to include 27 institutes and centers focusing on different aspects of health and medicine. The goals of the NIH are to foster creative scientific discoveries to advance the nation's ability to protect and improve health, to develop scientific knowledge and resources to prevent disease, to enhance the nation's economic well being by expanding our knowledge of medical science, and promote scientific integrity and social responsibility in scientific research conduct. The NIH maintains a comprehensive Web site with health information, grant opportunities, current research, and current news. The NIH also provides this information in English and Spanish, has freely available and downloadable audio reports concerning health information, and provides a number of multimedia options for sharing information including video and image galleries. A vast array of information on autism is available through the NIH for parents, professionals, and researchers.

National Institutes of Neurological Disorders and Stroke (NINDS)

Web site: http://www.ninds.nih.gov/

The mission of the NINDS is to reduce the burden of neurological disease. The NINDS supports and conducts basic and clinical research on the normal and diseased nervous system, supports training and education in the basic and clinical neurosciences, and aims to increase understanding and effectiveness of the diagnosis, treatment, and prevention of neurological disorders. Basic research concerns research that provides insight into a disorder, such as work with brain cells, the nervous system, or genetics. Clinical research concerns research that provides insight into a clinical disorder or insight into the treatment, prevention, or cure of a disorder through work with individuals with the disorder. Clinical research might be a clinical trial of a medication or the use of imaging work to examine how the brain of an individual with a disorder functions while performing a specific task. Both aspects of research into neuroscience are needed to impact our understanding of neurological disorders. The institute maintains a Web site with health information concerning neurological disorders, including autism; patient resources, publications in both English and Spanish; research opportunities for families and scientists, as well as training opportunities for professionals working in the field of neurological disorders.

National Institutes on Deafness and Other Communication Disorders (NIDCD)

Web site: http://www.nidcd.nih.gov/about/

The NIDCD is an institute of the National Institutes of Health established in 1988 that conducts and supports research that focuses on the normal and disordered processes of hearing, balance, smell, taste, voice, speech and language. Areas of focus include research on biomedical and behavioral problems associated with individuals who have communication impairments or disorders. The institute maintains a Web site with information on communication and communication disorders, balance, hearing and deafness, as well as smell and taste. In addition to specific health information, free publications, a directory of related organizations, links to other resources, and educational materials are available through the institute. The NIDCD maintains a Web page focusing on autism, including information about the disorder, links to other resources, and current research on the disorder.

National Institutes on Disability and Rehabilitation Research (NIDRR)

Web site: http://www.ed.gov/about/offices/list/osers/nidrr/index.html

The NIDRR is a division of the Office of Special Education and Rehabilitative Services in the U.S. Department of Education. The NIDRR focuses on research into the rehabilitation of individuals with disabilities. The institute provides leadership and support for a comprehensive program of research with an aim to improve the lives of individuals with disabilities from birth through adulthood. The organization generates and publishes materials regarding disability, including summaries of research and survey results; maintains a number of databases regarding disability, such as databases regarding traumatic brain injury and developmental disabilities; and provides information regarding legislation, policy, and research concerning disabilities. All research findings from the NIDRR are collected and disseminated the National Rehabilitation Information Center (NARIC).

National Library of Medicine

Web site: http://www.nlm.nih.gov/

The National Library of Medicine is the world's largest medical library and is a project of the National Institutes of Health. The library collects materials and provides information in all areas of biomedicine and health care. Through the library's Web site, viewers can access a number of databases and resources including (among others):

Pubmed: a searchable database of scientific publications in the biomedical literature. http://www.ncbi.nlm.nih.gov/sites/entrez. An entry of "autism" returns 14,616 entries.

MedlinePlus: health and drug information for patients and families (in English and Spanish). Autism: http://www.nlm.nih.gov/medlineplus/autism.html.

Genetics Home Reference: information regarding genetic conditions presented in everyday language. http://ghr.nlm.nih.gov/.

U.S. Department of Health and Human Services (HHS)

Web site: http://www.hhs.gov/

The U.S. Department of Health and Human Services (HHS) is the federal government's primary agency focused on the protection of health of all Americans and the provision of essential human services, especially for those who are least able to help themselves. The work of HHS is conducted by the 11 agencies under its arm, including the Centers for Disease Control and Prevention and National Institutes of Health. Through the 300 plus programs supported by HHS, the department supports research and federal services focusing on health and protecting the health of all Americans. HHS maintains an autism specific Web site with information for families and professionals: http://www.hhs.gov/autism/.

University-Based Organizations

Autism Center of Excellence and Healthy Infant Development Lab, University of California–San Diego

Web site: http://www.autismsandiego.org/

The Autism Center of Excellence and Healthy Infant Development Lab is based at the University of California–San Diego and was established under the direction of Eric Courchesne, PhD. The program is "dedicated to understanding how brain structure and function contribute to the health and well-being of all children" and focused on exploring the causes of autism using a multidisciplinary research approach. The center maintains a Web site with information regarding autism spectrum disorders, the research being conducted by the faculty and affiliates of the center, as well as information for parents, professionals, and students interested in becoming involved with the center.

Autism Intervention Research Program, University of California–San Diego

Web site: http://autismlab.ucsd.edu/

The Autism Intervention Research Program based at the University of California, San Diego (UCSD) was established by Laura Schreibman, PhD, and has been in existence since 1984. This research program focuses on the experimental analysis and treatment of autism, primarily the development and evaluation of Pivotal Response Training (PRT), an empirically supported, naturalistic, behaviorally based intervention program.

Drexel Autism Center

Web site: http://www.drexelmed.edu/Home/
AboutTheCollege/DepartmentsCentersandInstitutes/Centers/
DrexelAutismCenter.aspx

The Drexel Autism Center, established by Richard Malone, MD, is based in the department of psychiatry at Drexel University College of Medicine. The interdisciplinary team includes child psychiatrists, a pediatric nurse practitioner, a psychologist and a pediatric neurologist. With a mission to "advance knowledge about autism through research and to provide services to affected children and their families," the center provides evaluation services for families and provides opportunities for families to participate in studies on autism treatment. In an effort to increase autism awareness, center staff and affiliates provide outreach in the form of educational programs to schools, community agencies and area hospitals.

Emory Autism Center

Web site: http://www.psychiatry.emory.edu/PROGRAMS/autism/

The Emory Autism Center opened in 1991 in a collaborative effort between the University and public and private entities and it is housed in the Department of Psychiatry and Behavioral Sciences at Emory University School of Medicine. The Emory Autism Center provides diagnosis, family support and innovative treatment, as well as professional training. The Emory Autism Center has a family support program, provides comprehensive medical care and diagnostic evaluations, provides interdisciplinary training, engages in research, and engages in community outreach. There is information available on the Emory Autism Center Web site concerning available research opportunities and clinical contact information.

Florida Atlantic University Center for Autism and Related Disabilities (CARD)

Web site: http://www.coe.fau.edu/card/

The Florida Atlantic University CARD is an outreach and support program for individuals with autism spectrum disorders and their families as well as the professionals working with them. The Florida Atlantic University CARD program is one of seven CARD program throughout Florida State funded by the Florida Legislature through the Florida Department of Education. Please see the University of Miami and Nova Southeastern University Center for Autism and Related Disorders (UM-NSU CARD) entry for information regarding the Florida CARD system. The Florida Atlantic University CARD catchment area consists of five counties near the Boca Raton area.

Florida State University Center for Autism and Related Disabilities (CARD)

Web site: http://autism.fsu.edu/

The Florida State University CARD is an outreach and support program for individuals with autism spectrum disorders and their families as well as the professionals working with them. The Florida State University CARD program is one of seven CARD program throughout Florida State funded by the Florida Legislature through the Florida Department of Education. Please see the University of Miami and Nova Southeastern University Center for Autism and Related Disorders (UM-NSU CARD) entry for information regarding the Florida CARD system. The Florida State University CARD catchment area consists of 18 counties near the Tallahassee area.

Indiana Resource Center for Autism (IRCA), Indiana University

Web site: http://www.iidc.indiana.edu/irca/fmain1.html

The IRCA is part of the Indiana Institute on Disability located at Indiana University. IRCA provides a number of services including: outreach training focusing on evidence-based practices for teaching, support, and treatment in the community, home and school; consultation services; training and support for school teams and programs; and information dissemination regarding autism spectrum disorders through individual requests and media including newsletters and the Web. Additionally, IRCA engages in research focusing on improving and enhancing treatment programming with an aim to inform policy and maintains a comprehensive database for use in research and program evaluation. The Web site provides information regarding these services and how to access them as well as information regarding autism spectrum disorders and specific Indiana State services.

Kennedy Krieger Institute Center for Autism and Related Disorders

Web site: http://www.kennedykrieger.org/kki_cp.jsp?pid=1394

The Center for Autism and Related Disorders (CARD) at Kennedy Krieger Institute is a multidisciplinary program for children with autism spectrum disorder and their family members. With a goal of improving the lives of individuals with ASD, their families, and their communities, CARD provides clinical services (both assessment and intervention), conducts research, and engages in community outreach. There are four primary programs at CARD, including the Clinical Program, providing evaluations and treatment; the Achievements Therapeutic Day Program, providing individualized care in a small group setting; the REACH Research Program, conducting multidisciplinary research in ASD; and Outreach and Training, which includes training for professionals and families. Information regarding the programs and services available through CARD at Kennedy Krieger is posted on the Web site. Links to other organizations and Web sites and current autism news updates are also available on the Web site.

Massachusetts General Hospital, Learning and Developmental Disabilities Evaluation and Rehabilitation Services (LADDERS)

Web site: http://www.ladders.org/

LADDERS is an interdisciplinary program directed by Margaret Bauman, MD, designed to provide services in the evaluation and treatment of children and adults with autism spectrum disorders. LADDERS is part of the Lurie Marks Autism Center at Massachusetts General Hospital and the organization's aim is to address the overall needs of the child and family members by establishing therapeutic and programmatic goals for each individual child from a multidisciplinary perspective. Services provided by LADDERS include diagnostic evaluations; medical, cognitive and behavioral interventions including speech and language; occupational and physical therapy; psychological evaluation and counseling; parent skills training and family empowerment; and referral support for additional resources. In addition to providing clinical services, LADDERS provides practicum opportunities for medical students and graduate students focusing on autism spectrum disorders and also engages in research in autism. Through the LADDERS Web site, information regarding the LADDERS clinical and research services, as well as information about upcoming events and autism in the news, is available.

Thompson Center for Autism and Neurodevelopmental Disorders, University of Missouri

Web site: http://thompsoncenter.missouri.edu/

The Thompson Center for Autism and Neurodevelopmental Disorders at the University of Missouri was established in 2005 and is the largest center in Missouri specializing in autism and other developmental disorders. The Thompson Center provides diagnostic, assessment and treatment services for children, youth and young adults with an emphasis on comprehensive individualized services including specialized medical, therapeutic, educational and behavioral interventions. The Thompson Center is also a training program for professionals and families and includes training for students at the University of Missouri. Additionally, faculty members at the Thompson Center conduct a range of research projects and programs focused on autism spectrum disorders.

Treatment and Education of Autistic and Related Communication-Handicapped Children (TEACCH) Program, University of North Carolina, Chapel Hill

Web site: http://www.teacch.com

TEACCH was established in the early 1970s by Eric Schopler, PhD, and is an evidence-based service, training, and research program for children and adults with autism spectrum disorders of all skill levels. The aims of the TEACCH approach are "skill development and fulfillment of fundamental human needs such as dignity, engagement in productive and personally meaningful activities, and feelings of security, self-efficacy, and self-confidence." Dr. Schopler and the TEACCH program developed the idea of the "culture of autism," which is way of conceptualizing the characteristic patterns of thinking and behavior of individuals with autism spectrum disorders. This culture of autism includes: a relative strength in and preference for processing visual information as opposed to challenges in processing auditory information and language; attention to details but challenges in integrating these details; difficulty combining ideas; challenges in organizing ideas, materials, and activities; attentional difficulties; communication problems; challenges with organizing time; a tendency to become attached to routines, which results in difficulties in generalizing learned skills; very strong interests; and marked sensory preferences and dislikes. Based on this culture of autism, TEACCH developed "Structured Teaching," an intervention approach in which an individualized, person and family centered plan is developed for each student, the physical environment is structured, and extensive visual supports are utilized to make the educational experience predictable and understandable. TEACCH maintains a Web site with information regarding autism spectrum disorders, services and resources in North Carolina, training opportunities, and links to related sites and resources.

University of California, Davis, Medical Investigation of Neurodevelopmental Disorders (M.I.N.D.) Institute

Web site: http://www.ucdmc.ucdavis.edu/mindinstitute/

The physicians and doctoral level clinicians at the M.I.N.D. Institute provide comprehensive clinical care and conduct research in neurodevelopmental disorders including attention deficit, hyperactivity disorder, autism spectrum disorder, and learning disorders. The research conducted at the M.I.N.D. Institute focuses on the multidisciplinary and collaborative investigation into neurodevelopmental disorders through integration of scientists in the biological, environmental, medical and toxicological sciences. The clinic provides diagnostic and evaluation services for neurodevelopmental disorders and employs professionals from the U.C. Davis Departments of Pediatrics, Neurology, and Psychiatry and Behavioral Sciences. The health care professionals represented at the clinic include: physicians, psychologists, occupational and speech therapists, nurses, social workers, and child life specialists. Education is a third component of the M.I.N.D. Institute. Year-round educational opportunities are available to the general public; professionals in K–12 education, professionals in the fields of psychology, neurology and related fields; and students completing undergraduate or graduate degrees regarding the assessment, diagnosis, and treatment of neurodevelopmental disorders. The M.I.N.D. Institute's Web site provides information regarding the available studies, clinical services, educational opportunities, and fact sheets focusing on specific neurodevelopmental disorders, including autism.

University of California, Los Angeles, Center for Autism Research and Treatment (CART)

Web site: http://www.autism.ucla.edu/index2.php

UCLA has a long history of autism research, beginning in the 1960s with Ivar Lovaas' work in the treatment of autism based on principles of applied behavioral analysis. The UCLA CART was established in 2003. With a focus on improving our understanding of the biological basis and neurobehavioral mechanisms of autism with a goal to identify and improve new and effective treatments for autism and autism spectrum disorders, CART is comprised of faculty members from the Semel Institute and the departments of Neurology, Genetics, Neurobiology and Psychology at UCLA. A key impetus for the interdisciplinary collaboration to establish CART was the National Institutes for Mental Health (NIMH) funded "Studies To Advance Autism Research and Treatment (STAART)" award that UCLA received. Prior to being the recipient of the STAART award, UCLA was one of the ten Collaborative Programs of Excellence in Autism (CPEA) funded by the National Institutes of Child Health and Human Development (NICHD). UCLA also became one of the Autism Centers of Excellence (ACE) funded by the National Institutes of Health (NIH) and was also a recipient of one of the Autism Centers of Excellence network awards. The primary focus of CART's research program into autism is the understanding and exploration of the origins of the social communicative deficits observed in autism spectrum disorders at the genetic, neurological and psychological level. A second area of focus is in the treatment of autism spectrum disorders. Finally, CART aims to provide outreach and education to professionals and families, create collaborations between professionals, and promote the exchange of ideas among scientists and practitioners regarding autism spectrum disorders. On the CART Web site information regarding specific research opportunities, clinical programs available at UCLA for the autism community, and events and news is available.

University of Central Florida Center for Autism and Related Disabilities (CARD)

Web site: http://www.ucf-card.org/

The University of Central Florida CARD is an outreach and support program for individuals with autism spectrum disorders and their families as well as the professionals working with them. The University of Central Florida CARD program is one of seven CARD program throughout Florida State funded by the Florida Legislature through the Florida Department of Education. Please see the University of Miami and Nova Southeastern University Center for Autism and Related Disorders (UM-NSU CARD) entry for information regarding the Florida CARD system. The University of Central Florida CARD catchment area consists of seven counties near the Orlando area.

University of Florida at Jacksonville Center for Autism and Related Disabilities (CARD)

Web site: http://www.hscj.ufl.edu/pediatrics/autism/

The University of Florida at Jacksonville CARD is an outreach and support program for individuals with autism spectrum disorders and their families as well as the professionals working with them. The University of Florida at Jacksonville CARD program is one of seven CARD program throughout Florida State funded by the Florida Legislature through the Florida Department of Education. Please see the University of Miami and Nova Southeastern University Center for Autism and Related Disorders (UM-NSU CARD) entry for information regarding the Florida CARD system. The University of Florida at Jacksonville CARD catchment area consists of six counties with the regional headquarters in Jacksonville.

University of Florida Center for Autism and Related Disabilities (CARD)

Web site: http://card.ufl.edu/

The University of Florida CARD is an outreach and support program for individuals with autism spectrum disorders and their families as well as the professionals working with them. The University of Florida CARD program is one of seven CARD program throughout Florida State funded by the Florida Legislature through the Florida Department of Education. Please see the University of Miami and Nova Southeastern University Center for Autism and Related Disorders (UM-NSU CARD) entry for information regarding the Florida CARD system. The University of Florida CARD catchment area consists of 14 counties near the Gainesville area.

University of Miami and Nova Southeastern University Center for Autism and Related Disorders (UM-NSU CARD)

Web site: http://www.umcard.org/

The UM-NSU CARD is an outreach and support program for individuals with autism spectrum disorders and their families as well as the professionals working with them. UM-NSU CARD is one of seven CARD program throughout Florida State funded by the Florida Legislature through the Florida Department of Education. UM-NSU CARD provides services that are free of charge in three Florida counties: Miami-Dade, Broward, and Monroe Counties. The other regional, nonresidential CARD programs are based at Florida State University, the University of Central Florida, the University of Florida at Gainesville, the University of Florida Health Science Center at Jacksonville, the University of South Florida, and Florida Atlantic University. CARD services include individual and family support, program consultation, parent and professional training, as well as public awareness and community outreach. These CARD services expand on the capacities of state and local resources, but are not in place to duplicate these services. Each CARD program is supervised by a board comprised of family members of individuals with autism who help direct the CARD program policy and priorities. The CARD program was established in 1993 following the passing of the statute authoring the program and providing start-up funds. This was the result of several years of legislative work. In 1987, the Florida Legislature authorized and funded a Task Force on Autism. This task force, based out of the Florida Mental Health Institute at the University of South Florida, produced a report in 1988 recommending the development of comprehensive, regional resource and training centers throughout Florida. Two years later, the state legislature and the

State's Department of Education funded a successful pilot project that led to the 1993 establishment of the seven CARD programs. The UM-NSU CARD Web site provides information regarding autism spectrum disorders (available in English, Spanish and Creole), the CARD program, services provided by UM-NSU CARD, available resources to individuals, families, and professionals, and links to other resources.

University of Michigan Autism and Communication Disorders Centers (UMACC)

Web site: http://www.umaccweb.com/

The UMACC is an academically based center with a mission to improve the lives of individuals with autistic spectrum disorders and their families. The center aims to achieve this mission through education, research, and the provision of clinical services. Educational opportunities include graduate and postdoctoral training experiences and specific training in the gold standard diagnostic instruments (Autism Diagnostic Interview—Revised, ADI & Autism Diagnostic Observation Schedule, ADOS) developed in part by the director of the center, Catherine Lord, PhD. The research focus at UMACC is on the etiology and course, as well as intervention and prevention, of autism spectrum disorders. UMACC is the lead site in the Simons Simplex Collection, the international collaboration to explore the genetics of autism, funded by the Simons Foundation. UMACC also provides clinical services to individuals, families and the community. These include diagnostic and evaluation services, early intervention, consultation services to schools and other professionals, and social skills groups. On the UMACC Web site, information regarding educational, clinical, and research opportunities are listed. Additionally, specific information regarding diagnostic instruments, links to other resources, and recommended readings are highlighted.

University of South Florida Center for Autism and Related Disabilities (CARD)

Web site: http://card-usf.fmhi.usf.edu/

The University of South Florida CARD is an outreach and support program for individuals with autism spectrum disorders and their families as well as the professionals working with them. The University of South Florida CARD program is one of seven CARD program throughout Florida State funded by the Florida Legislature through the Florida Department of Education. Please see the University of Miami and Nova Southeastern University Center for Autism and Related Disorders (UM-NSU CARD) entry for information regarding the Florida CARD system. The University of South Florida CARD catchment area consists of 14 counties near the Tampa area.

University of Washington Autism Center

Web site: http://depts.washington.edu/uwautism/

Established by Geraldine Dawson, PhD, in 2001, the University of Washington Autism Center has focused on providing clinical and training services and conducting cutting edge research into autism spectrum disorders. The mission of the UW Autism Center is to "provide state-of-the-art clinical services, increase capacity for services through training, increase knowledge and awareness about autism in the professional community and general public, and conduct research aimed at improving the lives of individuals with autism and their families." The UW Autism Center is a component of the Center on Human Development and Disability at the University of Washington and includes faculty and staff from the University of Washington School of Medicine, College of Arts and Sciences, and College of Education. The clinical arm of the UW Autism Center provides diagnostic evaluations and multi-disciplinary intervention services for children with autism spectrum disorders from infancy through adolescence. The clinic team also offers a wide range of professional training opportunities. The research arm of the UW Autism Center has a long history of federal and private funding focused on increasing knowledge regarding the early diagnosis of autism; the neurobiological basis of autism; brain functioning, language, and cognitive development in autism; early biological and behavioral predictors of outcome; the genes related to autism; and behavioral and biological treatments for autism. Under Dr. Dawson's leadership, the UW Autism Center was one of the ten Collaborative Programs of Excellence in Autism (CPEA) funded by the National Institutes of Child Health and Human Development (NICHD). Similarly, the UW Autism Center was one of the sites in the National Institutes for Mental Health's (NIMH)

"Studies To Advance Autism Research and Treatment (STAART)" collaboration. The UW Autism Center also became one of the Autism Centers of Excellence (ACE) funded by the National Institutes of Health (NIH) in 2007. In January 2008, Dr. Dawson accepted a position at Autism Speaks, becoming Professor Emeritus at the University of Washington, at which she had a professor since 1985. Wendy Stone, PhD, accepted a position in 2009 as the new executive director of the UW Autism Center.

Yale Autism Program

Web site: http://www.info.med.yale.edu/chldstdy/autism

The Yale Autism Program, based at the Yale Child Study Center, is an interdisciplinary collaboration of scientists and clinicians focused on the provision of comprehensive clinical services to children with autism spectrum disorders and their families and conducting cutting-edge research. Directed by Ami Klin, PhD, the Yale Autism Program was established as one of the National Institutes of Health Autism Center of Excellence. The clinical and research programs involve infants, toddlers, preschool, and school-age children, and young adults with autism. Faculty and staff at the Yale Autism Program include professionals from the fields of clinical psychology, neuropsychology, neuroimaging, child psychiatry, speech-language pathology, social work, genetics and the biological sciences, psychopharmacology and psychiatric nursing. The Yale Autism Program maintains a Web site that contains information regarding autism spectrum disorders, available clinical and research-based services and opportunities, and links to resources for families and professionals. The Yale Child Study Center, of which the Yale Autism Program is a component, has been in existence since the early 1900s and is currently directed by Fred Volkmar, MD. The Yale Child Study Center provides clinical services, training and education, community services, social policy advancement, and conducts research in all aspects of childhood mental health, including autism.

8

Resources

The following is intended to be a guide for key journal articles, books, videos, Internet Web sites, and other resources that may be helpful in learning more about ASDs. The list is organized by the type of resource and subject matter. There are new resources, agencies, books, and tools being developed daily about ASD. Therefore, this list is not meant to represent a complete resource guide or an exhaustive list of all the available autism resources. Rather, it serves as a sample of possible resources that may be useful for acquiring more information about ASD.

Print Resources

General Information about ASDs

Key Journal Articles

Dawson, Geraldine, Sara Webb, Gerard Schellenberg, Stephen Dager, Seth Friedman, Elizabeth Aylward, and Todd Richards. 2002. "Defining the Broader Phenotype of Autism: Genetic, Brain, and Behavioral Perspectives." *Developmental Psychopathology* 14 (3): 581–611.

This very comprehensive review article provides up-to-date information about our current knowledge of ASD in terms of genetic, cognitive neuroscience, animal, and clinical studies. Candidates for broader traits that are affected in ASD are offered: face processing, social affiliation or sensitivity to social reward, motor imitation ability, memory, executive function, and language ability.

Frith, Uta, and Francesca Happé. 1994. "Autism: Beyond 'Theory of Mind.'" *Cognition* **50 (1–3): 115–32.**

The theory of mind account of ASD dominated the field for many years and successfully predicted many impairments in socialization, imagination, and communication in the ASD population. However, a number of exceptions have emerged, such as consistent passing of tasks purported to test theory of mind and deficits in other nonsocial areas. In response to these exceptions, the authors present an alternative and perhaps complementary theory to explain the multitude of differences in individuals with ASD: the central coherence theory. This theory suggests that impairments in ASD are the result of increased attention to details and a limited ability to process context, resulting in a limited ability to understand the "big picture."

Rogers, Sally J., and Bruce Pennington. 1991. "A Theoretical Approach to the Deficits in Infantile Autism." *Development and Psychopathology* **3 (2): 137–62.**

This theoretical article suggests that early social abilities involving imitation, emotion sharing, and theory of mind are the primary deficits in ASD. They posit that these skills are foundational in developing social representations of self and other people. The involvement of the prefrontal cortex and executive function capacities are suggested to be the brain regions primarily involved in these deficits.

Books

Baron-Cohen, Simon, and Patrick Bolton. 1993. *Autism: The Facts.* **New York: Oxford University Press.**

Baron-Cohen and Bolton have written this book primarily for parents, but information covered may also be helpful for professionals. It serves as a general introduction to ASD and covers areas such as recognition of symptoms and diagnosis, causes, and treatments/educational techniques.

Frith, Uta. 1991. *Autism and Asperger Syndrome.* **Cambridge, UK: Cambridge University Press.**

Frith explores Asperger's Disorder, referring back to and including translations of Hans Asperger's original work and papers. Although Asperger published in the 1940s, his work is still applicable today, and Frith attempts to link his classic work with current issues. She provides clinical accounts of individuals with Asperger's Disorder as well as preliminary research data.

Klass, Perri, and Eileen Costello. 2003. *Quirky Kids: Understanding and Helping Your Child Who Doesn't Fit In.* **New York: Ballantine Books.**

Children with ASD are often described as "quirky." This book is helpful to parents of quirky children—both with and without ASD. Parents will benefit from increased insight into their children. Nice discussions of treatment options and intervention strategies in a variety of environments (e.g. home, groups, playgrounds) are also offered.

Klin, Ami, and Fred Volkmar. 2000. *Asperger Syndrome.* **New York: Guilford Press.**

Definitive information about Asperger's Disorder is covered in depth in this book. Perspectives from prominent researchers and clinicians with extensive expertise in Asperger's Disorder are combined into a readable comprehensive text. In addition to extensive information from professionals, parent essays are also included to exemplify the family experience of life with a child with Asperger's Disorder.

Kutscher, Martin. 2005. *Kids in the Mix of ADHD, LD, Asperger's, Tourette's, Bipolar, and More! The One Stop Guide for Parents, Teachers, and Other Professionals.* **London: Jessica Kingsley Publishers.**

Children can collect a multitude of diagnoses as they move through elementary and middle school. This book describes the often co-existing neurobehavioral disorders beginning in childhood, including autism, Asperger's Disorder, bipolar disorder, ADHD, learning disabilities, and depression. Through case vignettes and practical advice, Kutscher describes the causes and symptoms of these disorders as well as their interactions with other conditions. Highly specific behavioral techniques are included that are effective for a variety of conditions.

Mesibov, Gary, Lynn Adams, and Laura Klinger. 1997. *Autism: Understanding the Disorder.* **New York: Plenum Press.**

The full range of current knowledge about ASD is included in this text, including history, diagnosis, causes, acting mechanisms, and treatment. Comprehensive and concisely written, it is appropriate for all audiences.

Neisworth, John, and Pamela Wolfe. 2005. *Autism Encyclopedia*. Baltimore, MD: Brookes Publishing Co.

This is a reference book that defines many terms associated with ASD. With approximately 500 entries, it provides a quick introduction to the field and its relevant areas, including therapies, diagnoses, and associated disorders. Complex concepts are defined clearly and concisely and can be easily understood by nonexperts.

Ozonoff, Sally, Geraldine Dawson, and James McPartland. 2002. *A Parent's Guide to Asperger Syndrome and High-Functioning Autism*. New York: Guilford Press.

This book provides information and advice for parents of children with Asperger's Disorder or high-functioning autism, including practical suggestions for successful life at home, school, and transition into adulthood. The authors emphasize using the individual's strengths to help him/her engage socially and live as self-sufficiently as possible. An exploration of scientific knowledge of autism is also included as well as real-life success stories and information on educational and life planning.

Powers, Michael. 2000. *Children with Autism: A Parent's Guide*. Rockville, MD: Woodbine House.

In this second edition, *Children with Autism* covers concerns specific to ASD, including daily and family life, early intervention, educational programs, legal rights, advocacy, and adulthood. Parent statements are provided at the end of each chapter to add a personal touch to the information described, and the reader benefits from this family perspective and support. Also translated into Spanish: Ninos Autistas: Guia para padres, terpeutas y educadores (Trillas 1999).

Schopler, Eric, Gary Mesibov, and Linda Kunce. 1998. *Asperger Syndrome or High-Functioning Autism?* New York: Springer.

The difference between Asperger's Disorder and high-functioning autism has been an area of controversy in the field for many years. This book explores current perspectives from experts about the disorders for the benefit of parents, teachers, and clinicians alike.

Sicile-Kira, Chantal, and Temple Grandin. 2004. *Autism Spectrum Disorders: The Complete Guide to Understanding Autism, Asperger's Syndrome, Pervasive Developmental Disorder, and Other ASDs.* New York: Penguin.

Sicile-Kira and Grandin describe the causes of ASD, discuss proper diagnostic procedures and treatments, offer coping strategies for families and advice about educational programs, and provide recommendations for living and working conditions for adults with ASD.

Stone, Wendy L., and Theresa Foy DiGeronimo. 2006. *Does My Child Have Autism: A Parent's Guide to Early Detection and Intervention in Autism Spectrum Disorders.* San Francisco: Jossey-Bass.

Stone and DiGeronimo intended this book to be a guide for parents to learn about early signs of ASD and early intervention services, prior to 2 years of age. The diagnostic process is described in detail, including what type of information parents will be expected to provide during the clinical evaluation. Intervention is also covered in depth, and the authors provide advice about obtaining the proper services for their children through doctors, counselors, therapists, and other professionals.

Szatmari, Peter. 2004. *A Mind Apart: Understanding Children with Autism and Asperger Syndrome.* New York: The Guilford Press.

Written with a positive outlook on ASD, Szatmari summarizes pressing concerns of parents of children with ASD and discusses current theories on causes, diagnosis, and treatment. The author presents the science of ASD in a respectful and easy-to-understand manner that many families will appreciate.

Volkmar, Fred, and Lisa Wiesner. 2009. *A Practical Guide to Autism: What Every Parent, Family Member, and Teacher Needs to Know.* Hoboken, NJ: John Wiley & Sons.

Volkmar and Wiesner, an autism scientist and pediatrician, teamed up to provide perspectives on the coordination of care for their child with autism in this book. Easy-to-access information is included about selection of professionals and services, and managing day-to-day life at home, in school, and elsewhere. General information about autism is also discussed.

Waltz, Mitzi. 1999. *Pervasive Developmental Disorders: Finding a Diagnosis and Getting Help for Parents and Patients with PDD-NOS and atypical PDD.* Arlington, TX: Future Horizons.

There are many books available for individuals with autism and Asperger's Disorder. However, there are limited resources geared specifically toward individuals with PDD-NOS, or atypical autism. This PDD-NOS guide helps parents to pursue a diagnosis for their child if they suspect they fit the category of PDD-NOS. Waltz describes effective treatments, ways of coping, and parent stories.

Wing, Lorna, Ami Klin, and Fred Volkmar. 2001. *The Autistic Spectrum: A Parents' Guide to Understanding and Helping Your Child.* Berkeley, CA: Ulysses Press.

Leaders in the field of autism have written this book for parents to better understand the oftentimes confusing disorder of ASD. The latest developments in the field are described as a means to understand ASD and improve upon communication and social interaction skills.

Wiseman, Nancy. 2006. *Could It Be Autism? A Parent's Guide to the First Signs and Next Steps.* New York: Random House.

Could It Be Autism? describes the red flags of ASD and early developmental concerns that may be indicative of ASD. The author is the founder of First Signs, which is an organization that is dedicated to the education of parents and professionals to help improve early detection of developmental disabilities. She is also the parent of a child with autism who was diagnosed early, and she shares her stories of success and challenge. Wiseman provides treatment recommendations that may be individualized to a child's particular developmental level.

Biological Mechanisms: Genetics and Neurological Functioning
Key Journal Articles
Bailey, Anthony, Anne Le Couteur, Irwin Gottesman, P. Bolton, E. Simonoff, E. Yuzda, and Michael Rutter. 1995. "Autism as a Strongly Genetic Disorder: Evidence from a British Twin Study." *Psychological Medicine* 25 (1): 63–77.

Bailey and colleagues reexamined the original twin pairs in Folstein and Rutter's (1977) study (described below) as well as 28 new autism twin pairs. They replicated the original paper's results suggesting increased likelihood of ASD in identical twin pairs as compared to fraternal twin pairs. Furthermore, they found that when they broadened the diagnostic boundaries of the disorder, the indication of genetic influence became even more prominent.

Baron-Cohen, Simon, Rebecca C. Knickmeyer, and Matthew K. Belmonte. 2005. "Sex Differences in the Brain: Implications for Explaining Autism." *Science* **310 (5749): 819–23.**

Baron-Cohen and colleagues present their "extreme male brain" theory positing that ASD represents an extreme form of a traditional male brain that, at a population level, is better at "systemizing" (e.g., operationalizing rules and systems and responding appropriately) than "empathizing" (e.g., inferring mental states and responding with appropriate emotions). The authors provide neuroanatomical findings to support this theory.

Courchesne, Eric, C. M. Karns, H. R. Davis, R. Ziccardi, R. A. Carper, Z. D. Tigue, H. J. Chisum, et al. 2001. "Unusual Brain Growth Patterns in Early Life in Patients with Autistic Disorder: An MRI Study." *Neurology,* **57 (2): 245–54.**

This study of brain volume and growth in very young children suggested that, on average, infants who went on to develop autism had normal brain volume at birth and then by 2–4 years of age had abnormally large brains as compared to typically developing children. This abnormality seemed to normalize by later childhood and adolescence, and brain volume was not significantly different from peers. Therefore, overall, findings suggested the presence of early overgrowth followed by abnormally slowed growth in children with autism.

Folstein, Susan, and Michael Rutter. 1977. "Infantile Autism: A Genetic Study of 21 Twin Pairs." *Journal of Child Psychology and Psychiatry* **18 (4): 297–321.**

This seminal article was the first to suggest that genetic factors are influential in the occurrence of ASD. Prior to the publication of this article, ASD was primarily thought to be a disorder caused by cold, aloof parenting. The authors found that identical twin pairs were significantly more likely to both have ASD as compared to fraternal twin pairs, suggesting that genetics play a strong role in the development of the disorder.

Schultz, Robert T. 2005. "Developmental Deficits in Social Perception in Autism: The Role of the Amygdala and Fusiform Face Area." *International Journal of Developmental Neuroscience* 23 (2–3): 125–41.

This article purposes that social deficits are primary in ASD, and Schultz provides neuroanatomical support for this theory. Specifically, he highlights early developmental problems with a brain region called the amygdala followed by cascading deficits in the development of cortical areas involved in visual social perception (i.e., the fusiform "face area" of the brain).

Sebat, Jonathan, B. Lakshmi, Dheeraj Malhotra, Jennifer Troge, Christa Lese-Martin, Tom Walsh, Boris Yamrom, et al. 2007. "Strong Association of De Novo Copy Number Mutations with Autism." *Science* 316 (5823): 445–49.

Findings from this ground-breaking genetics article suggested that the genetic causes of familial autism (i.e., families with more than one member with ASD) may differ from sporadic autism (i.e., families without a family history of ASD). Genetic mutations called de novo copy number variations (CNVs) were more likely to occur in the latter family type (simplex) as compared both to the former (multiplex) and families without a child with ASD.

General Intervention

Key Journal Articles

Lovaas, O. Ivar. 1987. "Behavioral Treatment and Normal Educational and Intellectual Functioning in Young Autistic Children." *Journal of Consulting and Clinical Psychology* 55 (1): 3–9.

In this seminal article, Lovaas reports on the outcomes of children with autism who received intensive behavioral intervention (called discrete trial training) as compared to those who did not receive it. Nearly half of the children in the intervention group achieved normal intellectual and educational functioning at treatment termination compared to very few in the nonintervention group. This was the first research study demonstrating that behavioral intervention can significantly improve outcomes for children on the spectrum.

McEachin, John J., Tristram Smith, and O. Ivar Lovaas. 1993. "Long-Term Outcome for Children with Autism who Received Early Intensive Behavioral Treatment." *American Journal on Mental Retardation* **97 (4): 359–72.**

In the follow-up article of Lovaas' original (1987) paper, the authors report that children who received study-administered behavioral intervention maintained their gains well into later childhood (~11.5 years). Those children with the most positive gains were indistinguishable from same-aged peers on tests of intelligence and adaptive behavior. Thus, this article demonstrated that behavioral treatment can produce lasting and substantial gains for some children with autism.

Books

Ball, James. 2008. *Early Intervention and Autism: Real-Life Questions, Real-Life Answers.* **Arlington, TX: Future Horizons.**

Ball describes necessary components to early intervention programs for young children with ASD and provides parents with the tools to decide which elements are essential for their child and family. Guides for setting up an Individual Family Service Plan (IFSP) are also discussed as well as tips for successful transitions to public school programs.

Dawson, Peg, and Richard Guare. 2004. *Executive Skills in Children and Adolescents: A Practical Guide to Assessment and Intervention.* **New York: Guilford Press.**

Children with ASD often struggle with tasks that require executive functioning. This guide provides a framework for strengthening such executive-functioning skills as planning, task initiation, and completion of homework on time. Environmental modifications are also discussed to help improve skills.

Dulcan, Mina K., and Tami Benton. 2007. *Helping Parents, Youth, and Teachers Understand Medications for Behavioral and Emotional Problems: A Resource Book of Medication Information Handouts (Second Edition).* **Arlington, VA: American Psychiatric Publishing.**

This book is composed of a series of practical handouts for parents, teachers, and children about medications prescribed for behavioral and emotional problems. The handouts are parent friendly and written in language that can be easily understood by the general public. Each handout has standardized information, including how the medication works, how long it lasts, and side effects and interactions with other medications and foods.

Greenspan, Stanley. 1997. *The Child with Special Needs: Encouraging Intellectual and Emotional Growth.* New York: Perseus Books.

Insight into many different kinds of special needs are covered in *The Child with Special Needs,* including autism, PDD, language and speech problems, Down syndrome, cerebral palsy, and ADD. Most of Greenspan's work is focused on the "what to do next" in moving forward with intervention capitalizing on a child's unique strengths and weaknesses. His well-known "floortime" model (using play techniques to improve developmental outcomes) is described in detail through direct instruction and case histories.

Harris, Sandra, and Mary Jane Weiss. 2007. *Right from the Start: Behavioral Intervention for Young Children with Autism.* Rockville, MD: Woodbine House.

Right from the Start is helpful for parents who are just beginning to explore the many intervention options available for their young children. The book provides discussions of various educational and treatment options available—from more naturalistic methods to structured teaching trials. Detailed background is provided for each type of intervention technique.

Koegel, Lynn Kern, and Claire LaZebnik. 2004. *Overcoming Autism.* New York: Viking Press.

An expert clinician/scientist and the parent of a child with ASD come together to offer ways to positively improve the life of a child with ASD. *Overcoming Autism* is a warm and nurturing book that uses a touch of humor to describe suggestions that can be easily adapted into a family's day-to-day life.

Koegel, Robert L., and Lynn Kern Koegel. 2005. *Pivotal Response Treatments for Autism.* Baltimore: Brookes Publishing.

The Koegels provide an in-depth exploration of Pivotal Response Treatment, an intervention that they developed to treat individuals with autism using naturalistic methods. This approach is described in detail in this updated and comprehensive book.

Koegel, Robert L., and Lynn Kern Koegel. 1995. *Teaching Children with Autism. Strategies for Initiating Positive Interactions and Improving Learning Opportunities.* **Baltimore: Brookes Publishing Co.**

The Koegels use a positive approach in this book to focus on how children with ASD *can* and *do* learn. Topics covered include behavioral characteristics of autism, intervention methods, long-term and short-term goals of intervention, and concrete suggestions for providing support to families.

Maurice, Catherine, Richard Foxx, and Gina Green. 2001. *Making a Difference: Behavioral Intervention for Autism.* **Austin, TX: Pro-Ed.**

In this follow-up volume of *Behavioral Intervention for Young Children* (1996), the editors combine data-based and scientific knowledge with practical, everyday tips for making informed decisions about the care for children with autism. Chapters written by parents provide personal insights into the intervention process. Additionally, professionals share their expertise about some creative strategies for working with children on the spectrum. Areas covered include eating, social skills, problem behaviors, promoting spontaneous language, prompting, and conversational skills, among many others.

Nowicki, Stephen, and Marshall P. Duke. 1992. *Helping the Child Who Doesn't Fit In.* **Atlanta: Peachtree Publishers.**

Many dimensions of childhood social rejection are analyzed, and difficulties with nonverbal communication are highlighted in *Helping the Child Who Doesn't Fit In.* The authors have created a term to describe the variety of difficulties common in ASD: *dyssemia,* meaning "difficulty with signals." Exercises for addressing dyssemia are provided, and guidance is offered for seeking professional help.

Richman, Shira. 2001. *Raising a Child with Autism: A Guide to Applied Behavior Analysis for Parents.* **London: Jessica Kingsley Publishers.**

Richman provides a comprehensive explanation of Applied Behavior Analysis (ABA), a method that has been effective in teaching children with ASD through behavior modification. The author explains how ABA can be used by parents at home to teach such skills as toilet training, self-dressing, communication, and addressing food selectivity.

Siegel, Bryna. 2003. *Helping Children with Autism Learn: Treatment Approaches for Parents and Professionals*. New York: Oxford University Press.

Helping Children with Autism Learn serves as a practical guide for addressing the learning challenges often associated with ASD. Instead of "symptoms," Siegel takes the unique approach that each child has a discrete set of "learning disabilities," each of which needs direct intervention. She offers advice for creating an educational program using proven techniques and emphasizes throughout the book the importance of having parents take the lead in their child's treatment.

Siegel, Bryna. 1996. *The World of the Autistic Child: Understanding and Treating Autistic Spectrum Disorders*. New York: Oxford University Press.

Siegel presents a complete guide to understanding and treating ASD. *The World of the Autistic Child* was one of the first truly comprehensive books about ASD and continues to be regarded as one of the most helpful books to empower parents to effectively manage their child's treatment program. Behavior modification, the development of daily living skills, psychoactive medications, residential placement, and schooling, including discussions about mainstreaming and effective parent-teacher relationships, are all covered.

Stewart, Kathryn. 2002. *Helping A Child with Nonverbal Learning Disorder or Asperger's Syndrome: A Parent's Guide*. Oakland, CA: New Harbinger Publications.

In her book, Stewart offers parents ways to help their child with challenges in such areas as visual and spatial functioning, writing, information processing and organization, social and emotional capabilities, and language.

Tsai, Luke. 2001. *Taking the Mystery Out of Medications in Autism/Asperger's Syndrome.* Arlington, TX: Future Horizons.

Although medication is not considered to be a first-line treatment for ASD, many families try medication at some point during the child's lifetime. Tsai discusses the variety of medications that parents of children with ASD might encounter and how they work in the body, including potential positive effects, side effects, and proper assessment of medication response.

Wilens, Timothy E. 2008. *Straight Talk about Psychiatric Medications for Kids.* New York: Guilford Publications.

The decision about moving forward with psychiatric medication for a child can be confusing and overwhelming for parents. This newly updated third edition discusses advances in medication treatment options and answers often-asked questions by parents: How do the medications work? How will it impact my child's emotions or personality? What are the risks? Many other areas are covered with updates about the latest developments in particular disorders.

Helpful Tools

Books

Baker, Bruce L., Jan B. Blacher, and Alan J. Brightman. 2003. *Steps to Independence: Teaching Everyday Skills to Children With Special Needs.* Baltimore: Brookes Publishing Co.

With more than 30 years of work with parents of children with special needs, the authors offer the fourth edition of the popular *Steps to Independence.* This hands-on resource provides parents with specific strategies needed for teaching independent living skills to children of all ages.

Baker, Jed, and Carol Stock Kranowitz. 2008. *No More Meltdowns: Positive Strategies for Managing and Preventing Out-of-control Behavior.* Arlington, TX: Future Horizons.

Baker's approach is based on years of applied research. Parents will learn the definition of a meltdown and why they are common in children. Importantly, the authors provide flexible strategies for how to manage these challenging behaviors.

Durand, Mark. 1998. *Sleep Better! A guide to Improving Sleep for Children with Special Needs*. Baltimore: Brookes Publishing Co.

Written by a psychologist who was inspired by many sleepless nights with his own child, *Sleep Better!* offers proven techniques to help improve sleep in children with special needs. Insights from the author's clinical and personal experience are included, making it a unique resource for both families and professionals.

Exkorn, Karen Siff. 2005. *The Autism Sourcebook: Everything You Need to Know about Diagnosis, Treatment, Coping and Healing*. New York: HarperCollins Publishers.

When Karen Siff Exhorn's son was diagnosed with autism, she had no information about the disorder. She educated herself quickly, and this book provides accessible medical information gleaned from the world's foremost experts. The author offers an inside look at families with children who have autism, tying in her own first-hand experience as a parent. *The Autism Sourcebook* is a comprehensive, practical resource available to parents and families of children with autism.

Gray, Carol. 2000. *The New Social Story Book Illustrated Edition*. Arlington, TX: Future Horizons.

Gray, the developer of social stories, offers 100 stories that offer explanations for what to do in everyday situations that children with ASD may find confusing. She details how to write a social story, so parents can tailor-make stories to fit their child's needs.

Hadwin, Julie, Simon Baron-Cohen, and Patricia Howlin. 1999. *Teaching Children With Autism to Mind-Read: A Practical Guide for Teachers and Parents*. Hoboken, NJ: John Wiley & Sons.

The authors explore the relationship between "theory of mind" deficits common in ASD and other areas of functioning. Detailed and practical guidelines are provided for specific teaching materials and strategies designed to help improve children's understanding of others' minds and points of view.

Hodgdon, Linda. 1999. *Solving Behavior Problems in Autism: Improving Communication with Visual Strategies*. Troy, MI: Quirk Roberts Publishing.

Solving Behavior Problems in Autism provides a practical approach to managing the complexity of behavior problems for children with ASD. Aimed at educators or parents who encounter children with behavior and self-management challenges, it is the second book in the Visual Strategies series and continues the approach of supporting communication with visual strategies.

Myles, Brenda, Catherine Cook, and Louanne Miller. 2000. *Asperger Syndrome and Sensory Issues: Practical Solutions for Making Sense of the World.* Shawnee Mission, KS: Autism Asperger Publishing Co.

This book uncovers the puzzling behaviors of children and youth with Asperger's Disorder that have a sensory base. Written in a reader-friendly style, the book offers a set of practical interventions that can be used by both parents and educators to help promote success for children and youth with Asperger's Disorder.

Myles, Brenda, and Jack Southwick. 1999. *Asperger Syndrome and Difficult Moments: Practical Solutions for Tantrums, Rage and Meltdowns.* Shawnee Mission, KS: Autism Asperger Publishing Co.

The expanded edition of this best-selling book offers parents and professionals alike effective solutions to handle "rage" in a child with Asperger's Disorder. Strategies to manage behaviors and reactions of adults around the child are also offered.

Notbohm, Ellen, and Veronica Zysk. 2004. *1001 Great Ideas for Teaching and Raising Children with Autism Spectrum Disorders.* Arlington, TX: Future Horizons.

In an easy-to-read format, the authors offer try-it-now solutions that have worked for thousands of children struggling with the social, sensory, behavioral, and self-care issues associated with ASD.

O'Neill, Robert, Robert Horner, Richard Albin, Keith Storey, and Jeffrey Sprague. 1996. *Functional Assessment and Program Development for Problem Behavior: A Practical Handbook.* Florence, KY: Wadsworth Publishing.

Readers of this guide will benefit from an introduction to functional assessment procedures, including ways to assess problem behaviors and tips about designing behavior programs based on the results of the assessments. Through these and other topics, the authors present methods for creating personalized intervention programs.

Quill, Kathleen Ann. 2000. *Do-Watch-Listen-Say: Social and Communication Intervention for Children With Autism.* **Baltimore: Paul H. Brookes Publishing.**

Backed by research-based methodology, this assessment and intervention guide offers educators hundreds of creative ideas to promote social and communication skills along with an assessment tool, the Assessment of Social and Communication Skills for Children with Autism. This tool contains a set of questionnaires and checklists that help to obtain a detailed profile of a child's abilities in more than 100 subskill areas. The book helps readers to target specific skills for intervention from which an individualized social and communication skills curriculum can be developed.

Savner, Jennifer, and Brenda Smith Myles. 2000. *Making Visual Supports Work in the Home and Community: Strategies for Individuals with Autism and Asperger Syndrome.* **Shawnee Mission, KS: Autism Asperger Publishing Co.**

This book shows parents how to make and use visual supports. Easy to read, it provides step-by-step directions and pictures that can be geared to individual children and their families.

Smith Myles, Brenda, Melissa L. Trautman, and Ronda L. Schelvan. 2004. *Hidden Curriculum: Practical Solutions for Understanding Unstated Rules in Social Situations.* **Shawnee Mission, KS: Autism Asperger Publishing Co.**

Individuals with ASD often have difficulty picking up on more subtle rules of social interactions. Although these skills come naturally to typically developing children, they can be difficult to teach to children with ASD. This book offers a curriculum with practical suggestions and advice for how to help individuals with ASD to navigate the unspoken social world.

Sonders, Susan Aud. 2003. *Giggle Time—Establishing the Social Connection: A Program to Develop the Communication Skills of Children With Autism, Asperger Syndrome and PDD.* **London: Jessica Kingsley Publishers.**

This book describes an effective technique to build simple interactive games to develop communication with children with limited language. The book is clearly written and illustrated with photo examples of real-life games.

Wheeler, Maria. 2007. *Toilet Training for Individuals with Autism or Other Developmental Issues, 2nd Edition.* **Arlington, TX: Future Horizons.**

Individuals with autism are known to have much difficulty with toilet training. This how-to guide offers highly effective strategies taking into account children with autism's sensitivities rather than pushing traditional methods. It provides more than 200 dos and don'ts and over 50 real-life examples.

Social and Communication Skills
Books
Antonello, Stephen. 1995. *Social Skills Development: Practical Strategies for Adolescents and Adults with Developmental Disabilities.* **New York: Simon & Schuster Adult Publishing Group.**

This comprehensive social skills guide provides a complete collection of topics and subskills to enhance social communication skills in teenagers and adults with ASD. The skills covered range from basic communication to more complex skills with modifications provided for more functionally impaired individuals. Case vignettes and rationales behind the skills are provided to fully prepare the instructor to teach the skill.

Baker, Jed. 2006. *The Social Skills Picture Book for High School and Beyond.* **La Vergne, TN: Ingram Publisher Services.**

Especially useful for visual learners, Baker's social skills book for teenagers offers pictures of students engaging in a range of social situations intended to teach by *showing* (not only telling). Social situations that are relevant to teenagers are included in this book such as going on a date, making friends, and interviewing. The consequences of using various skills are also depicted to allow teens to begin to see the potential outcomes (both positive and negative) of their behavior during social interactions.

Baker, Jed. 2001. *The Social Skills Picture Book: Teaching Play, Emotion, and Communication to Children with Autism.* **Arlington, TX: Future Horizons.**

A well-known writer and expert in social skills training for individuals with autism, Baker offers this book as a means to teach youngsters with ASDs social skills appropriate during conversations, play, expressing emotions, and developing empathy. His pictures show the right and wrong ways to handle situations involving the use of these skills.

Baker, Jed. 2003. *Social Skills Training for Children and Adolescents with Asperger Syndrome and Social-Communication Problems.* **Shawnee Mission, KS: Autism Asperger Publishing Co.**

In another of Baker's popular books, he offers a proven social skills curriculum with ready-to-use activities appropriate for children with Asperger's Disorder of a variety of ages. Baker covers 70 skills that are often impacted in children with ASD via lessons with associated handouts and activity sheets describing ways to teach that particular skill, both in the classroom and at home.

Duke, Marshall P., Stephen Nowicki, and Elisabeth A. Martin. 1996. *Teaching Your Child the Language of Social Success.* **Atlanta: Peachtree Publishers.**

Teaching Your Child the Language of Social Success is intended to describe ways to teach *nonverbal* communication, such as gestures, facial expressions, and tone of voice. The rules of nonverbal communication are explained and broken down to help make this unspoken aspect of communication explicit through case studies, illustrations, and exercises appropriate for home or in the classroom.

Frankel, Fred. 1996. *Good Friends Are Hard to Find: Help Your Child Find, Make and Keep Friends.* **Glendale, CA: Perspective Publishing.**

Good Friends Are Hard to Find is intended to help children 5 to 12 years old learn to make friends and problem-solve social conflicts with peers using clinically tested methods that the author helped to develop. Frankel recommends one-on-one playdates as the best method to develop friendship skills and establish relationships. Concrete guidance on how to manage teasing and bullying is also provided.

Freeman, Sabrina, and Lorelei Dake. 1997. *Teach Me Language: A Language Manual for Children with Autism, Asperger's Syndrome* *and Related Developmental Disorders.* **Langley, British Columbia: SKF Books.**

Teach Me Language is a step-by-step manual intended to be a complete resource for teaching language to children with ASD. Speech pathology methods including instructional lessons, examples, explanations, and games/activities are provided to make learning as fun as possible while still teaching necessary skills. Areas targeted include social language, grammar and syntax, writing, and language-based academic concepts.

Grandin, Temple, and Sean Barron. 2005. *Unwritten Rules of Social Relationships: Decoding Social Mysteries through the Unique Perspectives of Autism.* Arlington, TX: Future Horizons.

Grandin and Barron, both successful adults with ASD, apply lessons they've learned in their lives to shed light into the complex and unspoken rules of social interactions and relationships. With an insider's view of living, working, and interacting with others as adults with ASD, they offer concrete guidelines and effective ways for others with ASD to navigate the social world.

Gray, Carol, and Abbie Leigh White. 2002. *My Social Stories Book.* London: Jessica Kingsley Publishers.

Social stories are narratives taking children step-by-step through a variety of basic activities. Gray created social stories as a means to teach social and life skills to children and lower functioning individuals with ASD. Social stories help prepare children on the spectrum for an upcoming new activity by making them comfortable with what to expect. This book contains over 200 social stories written for children aged 2–6 about a range of activities such as brushing your teeth and wearing a seatbelt.

Heinrichs, Rebekah. 2003. *Perfect Targets: Asperger Syndrome and Bullying: Practical Solutions for Surviving the Social World.* Shawnee Mission, KS: Autism Asperger Publishing Company.

The unique behaviors and characteristics of students with high-functioning autism and Asperger's Disorder often make them easy targets for bullying and teasing. This book examines bullying in the ASD population and offers adults specific interventions to address bullying and teasing in the hopes of preventing the long-term effects that repeated bullying often has on children.

Hodgdon, Linda. 1995. *Visual Strategies for Improving Communication: Practical Supports for School and Home.* **Troy, MI: Quirk Roberts Publishing.**

This is a comprehensive book explaining the use of visual strategies to help improve communication in students with autism and other related disorders. Practical ideas and techniques for creating solutions to communication challenges are included as well as many illustrated visual supports. Focus is placed both on understanding and expressing language relevant to a child's day-to-day life.

McAfee, Jeanette. 2002. *Navigating the Social World: A Curriculum for Individuals with Asperger's Syndrome, High Functioning Autism, and Related Disorders.* **Arlington, TX: Future Horizons.**

As a parent of a child diagnosed with Asperger's Disorder, pediatrician Jeanie McAfee created this user-friendly social curriculum for both parents and educators. McAfee covers how to increase communication skills, cope with emotions, recognize and prevent stress, develop abstract thinking skills, address behavioral problems, and other areas.

Quill, Kathleen. 1995. *Teaching Children with Autism: Strategies to Enhance Communication and Socialization.* **Albany, NY: Delmar Cengage Learning.**

Intended primarily for speech and language pathologists, this book is designed to promote communication and socialization in children with autism. Strategies and adaptations to traditional therapeutic interventions are included in such areas as communication in nonverbal children, play, reading social cues, and developing appropriate environmental supports.

Weiss, Mary Jane, and Sandra Harris. 2001. *Reaching Out, Joining In: Teaching Social Skills to Young Children with Autism.* **Rockville, MD: Woodbine House.**

Reaching Out, Joining In is intended for parents to use as a guide for teaching social skills to their young children (preschool through early elementary years) with ASD. The primary means of teaching skills is through Applied Behavioral Analysis with a focus on the following four areas: play, social language, taking another person's point view, and successful integration into an inclusive classroom. The programs described in this book build on a child's strengths using strategies such as games, videos, modeling, and rewards.

School and Education

Books

Blenk, Katie, and Doris Fine. 1994. *Making School Inclusion Work: A Guide to Everyday Practices.* Brookline, MA: Brookline Books.

Inclusive school programs can seem daunting to develop and maintain. The authors share their how-to strategies for developing truly inclusive school programs that welcome students of a variety of economic levels, ethnic and racial backgrounds, and ability levels. With respect to autism, the authors relay specifics about how to meet the needs of children with mild to serious special education needs in order to maximize benefit for *all* children in the classroom. Anecdotes of experiences from both typically developing and children with special needs and their parents are shared in *Making School Inclusion Work.*

Fouse, Beth. 1999. *Creating a Win Win IEP for Students with Autism.* Arlington, TX: Future Horizons.

Creating a Win Win IEP for Students with Autism is an introductory text for parents navigating the special educational system and learning to understand the Individualized Education Program (IEP) process. An introduction into "what is an IEP" and the legal background behind the necessity of IEPs are discussed. Acronyms and the special language of the educational world are explained in detail so that parents can be fully equipped to be knowledgeable and crucial members of their child's IEP team. Form letters are also included as well as discussions of teacher's legal responsibilities and family's rights.

Fullerton, Ann. 1996. *Higher Functioning Adolescents and Young Adults with Autism: A Teacher's Guide.* Austin, TX: Pro-Ed.

Higher Functioning Adolescents and Young Adults with Autism is geared toward high school teachers supporting students with autism. Emphasis is placed on issues particular to adolescence, including peer relations and establishing an adult identity. Some strategies offered may also be applicable for students of all grades.

Gibb, Gordon, and Tina Taylor Dyches. 2007. *Guide to Writing Quality Individualized Education Programs, 2nd Edition.* **Columbus, OH: Allyn & Bacon.**

This guide offers seven basic steps to writing an IEP based on the requirements of IDEA 2004. Its audience is teachers who are learning or fine-tuning their IEP-writing skills. Case studies are provided along with examples of complete IEPs for children of a variety of ages and ability levels. Step-by-step instruction for IEP development is also included via written explanation, models, and practice appropriate for group or individual learning.

Handleman, Jan, and Sandra Harris. 2008. *Preschool Education Programs for Children with Autism, 3rd Edition.* **Austin, TX: Pro-Ed.**

Preschool Education Programs for Children with Autism contains expert contributions from many national autism educational programs in addressing pertinent questions about the treatment and preschool education of very young children with autism. A variety of educational settings (e.g., public, private, and university-based programs) and topics are included, such as play, social skills, speech and language, visual supports, sign language, and transitioning to elementary school programs.

Mayerson, Gary. 2004. *How To Compromise With Your School District Without Compromising Your Child: A Field Guide for Getting Effective Services for Children with Special Needs.* **New York: DRL Books.**

Mayerson is a lawyer who has devoted his career to representing and advocating for children with autism to receive fair and appropriate education. He spells out the "must dos" and "must don'ts" for parents to follow when seeking special services from the educational system, including how to prepare for an IEP meeting, next steps when children are not receiving the services they need, and how to avoid invoking due process of law in ensuring proper educational services for children in need.

Reif, Sandra, and Julie Heimburge. 2006. *How to Reach and Teach All Children in the Inclusive Classroom: Practical Strate-*

gies, Lessons, and Activities, 2nd Edition. Hoboken, NJ: John Wiley & Sons.

A team approach to "reach and teach" all students in an inclusive classroom setting is described in *How to Reach and Teach All Children in the Inclusive Classroom.* The authors provide strategies, ready-to-use lesson plans, and activities for students with varied learning styles, ability levels, and behaviors. Teachers of grades 3–8 would maximally benefit from this book.

Siegel, Lawrence. 2009. *The Complete IEP Guide: How to Advocate for Your Special Ed Child, 6th Edition.* **Berkeley, CA: NOLO.**

The IEP is a key component in determining the special education services that children with autism will receive in school. *The Complete IEP Guide* helps reader to sift through the paperwork and bureaucracy often associated with the IEP to put programs and school interventions into place to better help children in need. Understanding children's rights, eligibility, assessments, IEP goals/ objectives, and programs and services are discussed in detail in this user-friendly guide.

Smith Myles, Brenda, and Richard Simpson. 2003. *Asperger Syndrome: A Guide for Educators and Parents.* **Austin, TX: Pro-Ed.**

In addition to a general introduction to Asperger's Disorder and family stories of living with a child with the diagnosis, *Asperger Syndrome: A Guide for Educators and Parents* offers educational strategies to help enhance students' learning. Interventions for home and school are discussed.

Turnbull, H. Rutherford, and Ann P. Turnbull. 2006. *Free Appropriate Public Education: The Law and Children with Disabilities, 7th Edition.* **Denver: Love Publishing Company.**

The Turnbulls are lawyers dedicated to representing families of children with special needs in the educational system. The latest edition of this reader-friendly textbook explains the often-complex legal process of special education. *Free Appropriate Public Education* is a crucial resource for parents and professionals who do not have access to training in the law behind special education. The text is broken into three parts: Introduction to the Law, the Principles of IDEA, and Enforcing the Law. Readers will learn about the history of IDEA and gain valuable information about using the law to obtain free appropriate education for children with special needs.

Wright, Pam, and Pete Wright. 2006. *From Emotions to Advocacy,* *2nd Edition.* **Boyne City, MI: Harbor House.**

The Wrights teach readers such strategies as planning, preparing, and organizing to better receive quality special education services for children in need. Worksheets, forms, and sample letters are included to help advocate for children's educational needs. Additionally, the potential for parent-school conflicts, the importance of paper trails, and effective letter-writing techniques are discussed.

Biography/Personal Stories/Stories
Books
Andron, Linda. 2001. *Our Journey through High Functioning Autism and Asperger Syndrome: A Roadmap.* London: Jessica Kingsley Publishers.

In this realistic and positive book, families of children with autism describe autism's impact on their lives and solutions to adapt successfully to the daily life challenges that arise. Strategies for helping children to develop empathy, humor, friendships, and share their diagnosis with others are described.

Barron, Judy, and Sean Barron. 2002. *There's a Boy in Here: Emerging from the Bonds of Autism.* **Arlington, TX: Future Horizons.**

This unique book is a dual autobiography written in point-counterpoint style by a mother of an individual with autism (Judy Barron) and her son (Sean Barron). The Barrons share the story of their lives, from a very difficult early childhood to a breakthrough that Sean experienced in his late teenage years. The combination of mother/son perspectives provides excellent insight into the full range of family impact of autism.

Grandin, Temple. 2006. *Thinking in Pictures: My Life with Autism.* **New York: Knopf Doubleday Publishing Group.**

In *Thinking in Pictures,* Grandin reveals her inner world as an individual with autism. She discusses how the thought processes of individuals with autism are different than those of the "outside world" and how she was able to move across this boundary to function in this world.

Grandin, Temple, and Margaret Scariano.1986. *Emergence: Labeled Autistic.* **New York: Warner Books.**

As discussed in Chapter 5 of this book, Grandin is a well-known woman and university professor diagnosed with autism at a young age. This firsthand account of Grandin's life tells the story of her life from early childhood when she was enrolled in a school for children with autism through adulthood. Grandin shares insight into the fears and feelings of isolation that many individuals with autism experience and offers theories and treatment modalities for families to try.

Haddon, Mark. 2003. *The Curious Incident of the Dog in the Nighttime.* **New York: Random House.**

The Curious Incident of the Dog in the Nighttime is a novel whose main character is Christopher Boone, a 15-year-old boy with Asperger's Disorder. Throughout the course of the book, Christopher investigates the murder of a neighborhood dog and overcomes some serious fears along his journey.

Hart, Charles. 1989. *Without Reason: A Family Copes with Two Generations of Autism.* **Arlington, TX: Future Horizons.**

Hart grew up living with his severely affected brother with autism. Later in life, Hart himself had a son with autism. This book is an account of Hart's life living with two generations of autism and his experience establishing accommodations for his son, brother, and others with disabilities to better allow them to be successful in the world. Hart's view is not to cure autism, but to understand and accommodate individuals with the disorder.

Jacobs, Barbara. 2004. *Loving Mr. Spock: Understanding an Aloof Lover.* **Arlington, TX: Future Horizons.**

Jacobs tells the story of her romantic relationship with Danny, a man with Asperger's Disorder. She compares Danny with "Mr. Spock" who often uses logic rather than emotion to guide his actions. Through personal experience, discussions of diagnostics, quotes from other couples, and more, Jacobs offers lessons for people who are in relationships with individuals on the spectrum and those on the spectrum themselves.

Maurice, Catherine. 1994. *Let Me Hear Your Voice: A Family's Triumph over Autism.* **New York: Random House Publishing.**

Let Me Hear Your Voice is a mother's account of her family's life and adjustment to autism. Maurice herself is the mother of a girl with autism who tells the story of her daughter's regression into autism during her second year of life and the subsequent journey of finding a treatment that worked. Eventually, her daughter made huge gains through behavioral intervention, called Applied Behavioral Analysis.

Newport, Jerry, and Mary Newport. 2007. *Mozart and the Whale: An Asperger's Love Story.* **New York: Simon & Schuster Adult Publishing Group.**

Jerry and Mary Newport share the story of their relationship as two geniuses with Asperger's Disorder who met and married. The couple became very well known, and they later divorced due to the stresses of being a public couple. Later in life, they remarried (each other) and, in this book, tell the story of their lives together and apart.

Park, Clara. 2002. *Exiting Nirvana: A Daughter's Life with Autism.* **New York: Back Bay Books.**

Park shares her experience of raising her daughter with autism in this moving book. Interwoven amongst her own life stories and those of her daughter are theories of autism and widespread thoughts about human nature in general.

Sanders, Robert. 2004. *On My Own Terms: My Journey with Asperger's.* **Murfreesboro, TN: Armstrong Valley Publishing.**

Sanders wrote this autobiography about living his life with Asperger's Disorder. He shares his experience through personal accounts, ideas for change, and insights into the disorder itself. Sanders now holds a degree in electrical engineering and has written several novels.

Shally, Celeste, and David Harrington. 2008. *Since We're Friends: An Autism Picture Book.* Centerton, AR: Awaken Specialty Press.

This illustrated story provides examples of how to make a friendship work with a child with ASD. The story is about two boys, one with autism and one without, who begin to develop a friendship. Young readers can learn that children with ASD can be fun and real partners in a friendship.

Welton, Jude. 2004. *Can I Tell You About Asperger Syndrome? A Guide for Friends and Family.* London: Jessica Kingsley Publishers.

Adam is a young man with Asperger's Disorder who tells his readers what it feels like to have Asperger's from his perspective. Children between 7 and 15 years of age would maximally benefit from this book to begin to understand differences and appreciate talents of children with Asperger's from a child's perspective.

Willey, Liane. *Asperger Syndrome in the Family: Redefining Normal.* London; Philadelphia: Jessica Kingsley Publishers, 2001.

Written by an individual with Asperger's Disorder (who also has a daughter with Asperger's), this book provides a personal account of the disorder. Willey offers abundant examples of practical hints for maximizing success for "Aspies" in social situations. She also includes information about resources and a different perspective about symptoms.

Willey, Liane. 1999. *Pretending to Be Normal: Living with Asperger's Syndrome.* London: Jessica Kingsley Publishers.

Pretending to be Normal is told through the eyes of Willey, a woman with Asperger's Disorder who came to accept and appreciate her personality after years of self-doubt and self-denial.

Williams, Sondra. 2005. *Reflections of Self.* Zeeland, MI: The Gray Center for Social Learning & Understanding.

Williams is the mother of four children with autism, married to a husband with autism, and has high-functioning autism herself. In *Reflections of Self,* she shares articles, poetry, and thoughts from her unique perspective and intimate relationship with autism.

Parenting/Family Issues/Parent Perspectives
Books

Fling, Echo. 2000. *Eating an Artichoke: A Mothers' Perspective on Asperger Syndrome*. London: Jessica Kingsley Publishers.

For much of her son's childhood, the author and her husband took their child to see a variety of doctors, specialists, and other professionals to learn what was different about their son. Fling finally received a diagnosis of Asperger's Disorder in her son at 10 years of age. In this book, Fling describes their journey and parent perspectives on the diagnosis.

Harris, Sandra. 2003. *Siblings of Children with Autism: A Guide for Families*. Rockville, MD: Woodbine House.

Siblings of children with ASD are a unique group of individuals—they are often strong supports for children on the spectrum and frequently take the backseat in family dynamics. *Siblings of Children with Autism* takes an in-depth look at the life of a sibling of a child with autism. It guides families through ways to explain the diagnosis to siblings, manage the sibling's own feelings, balance family needs, and prepare adult siblings for helping to manage the care of adults with ASD.

Johnston-Tyler, Jan. 2007. *The Mom's Guide to Asperger Syndrome and Related Disorders*. Shawnee Mission, KS: Autism Asperger Publishing Co.

This guide provides detailed and practical information for parents of children with Asperger's Disorder and other ASDs in seeking appropriate services and getting the help that parents need. Written by a parent of a child with Asperger's, *The Mom's Guide to Asperger Syndrome and Related Disorders* uses parent-friendly language and is intended to be a valuable resource throughout a child's lifetime.

Schopler, Eric. 1995. *Parent Survival Manual: A Guide to Crisis Resolution in Autism and Related Developmental Disorders*. New York: Plenum Press.

In this unique book, 350 parent stories have been compiled to serve as practical guides to managing a variety of challenging behaviors associated with ASD. Topics covered include aggression, commu-

nication, play and leisure, perseveration, eating, sleeping, and toi-
leting and hygiene. Behavior therapists have analyzed all anecdotes, and the stories serve as a quick reference for parents dealing
with similar issues at home.

Books for Individuals with Autism

Books

Dunn Buron, Kari. 2003. *When My Autism Gets Too Big! A Relaxation Book for Children with Autism Spectrum Disorders* (also
called *When My Worries Get Too Big! A Relaxation Book for Children Who Live with Anxiety*). Shawnee Mission, KS: Autism Asperger Publishing Co.

"Losing control" is an often-reported concern of both parents and
individuals with ASD. In this illustrated book, relaxation techniques are introduced and taught as a way to manage feelings when
children begin to feel out of control.

Edwards, Andreanna. 2002. *Taking Autism to School*. Plainview,
NY: JayJo Books.

This illustrated storybook is intended to teach young children about
the daily lives of children with autism. It is helpful in encouraging
peers to better understand the particular differences common in
children with ASD, with the goal of allowing peers to better empa-
thize with them.

Faherty, Catherine. 2000. *Aspergers . . . What Does It Mean to Me?*
Arlington, TX: Future Horizons.

This workbook is intended for children with high-functioning autism or Asperger's Disorder in order to learn more about themselves. Children can write in the book and respond to a variety of
subjects that Faherty offers. Pages can be easily photocopied.

Vermuelen, Peter. 2000. *I Am Special: Introducing Children and
Young People to their Autistic Spectrum Disorder.* London: Jessica
Kingsley Publishers.

This child-friendly workbook is designed for a child with ASD
to fill out with an adult. It introduces the child to their diagnosis

through worksheets, exercises, and the creation of a personal book about themselves. Strengths of individuals of ASD are highlighted, and children are encouraged to view their differences positively.

Adolescence
Books
Newport, Jerry, and Mary Newport. 2002. *Autism-Asperger's and Sexuality: Puberty and Beyond*. Arlington, TX: Future Horizons.

A husband and wife who are both diagnosed with Asperger's Disorder have written this book to provide advice on dating, sex, birth control, disease prevention, abuse, and personal responsibility in day-to-day life and relationships. Discussions on how to develop loving relationships with sexual intimacy are also covered.

Nichols, Shana. 2008. *Girls, Growing Up on the Autism Spectrum: What Parents and Professionals Should Know about the Pre-teen and Teenage Years*. London: Jessica Kingsley Publishers.

One of the few pieces of work specifically geared toward teenage girls with ASD, *Girls, Growing Up on the Autism Spectrum* covers areas of concern commonly reported to be difficult for adolescent girls on the spectrum. Topics include fitting in with peers, friendships, and physical changes associated with puberty (e.g., starting your period). The authors provide knowledge and advice families need to successfully navigate the teenage years through professional expertise and family stories.

Sicile-Kira, Chantel. 2006. *Adolescents on the Autism Spectrum: A Parent's Guide to the Cognitive, Social, Physical, and Transition Needs of Teenagers with Autism Spectrum Disorders*. New York: A Perigee Book.

This book is geared to the needs of preteens and teenagers with ASD ranging from mildly to severely impaired. Cognitive, emotional, social, and physical needs are covered in depth using case examples and practical advice. New areas of focus that emerge in adolescence are also covered, including increased risk of seizures, understanding sexuality and dating, and preparing for life after high school.

Smith Myles, Brenda, and Diane Adreon. 2001. *Asperger Syndrome and Adolescence: Practical Solutions for School Success.* **Shawnee Mission, KS: Autism Asperger Publishing Company.**

Transition to middle and high school can be an emotional and traumatic time for teenagers with Asperger's Disorder. This book includes an in-depth exploration about why teens with Asperger's are at particular risk for such challenges. Helpful supports and strategies are also provided to make the transition smoother for teens and to maximize success at school.

Wrobel, Mary. 2003. *Taking Care of Myself: A Healthy Hygiene, Puberty and Personal Curriculum for Young People with Autism.* **La Vergne, TN: Ingram Publisher Services.**

Written by a speech and language pathologist, this book provides a variety of lessons for individuals with ASD to guide children and caregivers through issues of health, hygiene, and puberty.

Adulthood

Books

Baker, Jed. 2006. *Preparing for Life: The Complete Guide for Transitioning to Adulthood for Those with Autism and Asperger's Syndrome.* **Arlington, TX: Future Horizons.**

In another of his best-selling books, Baker covers "Life Skills Training" in this book to help individuals with ASD be successful after high school. Topics covered include lessons on nonverbal cues (e.g., body language), how to deal with emotions, and tips on friendships and intimate relationships. Laws regarding accommodations for adults with disabilities are also discussed.

Grandin, Temple, and Kate Duffy. 2008. *Developing Talents: Careers for Individuals with Asperger Syndrome and High-Functioning Autism.* **Shawnee Mission, KS: Autism Asperger Publishing Co.**

This book is intended to explore career options for adults with ASD. The authors highlight the growing number of career opportunities in entrepreneurship (among other fields) in today's society that are well suited for the unique characteristics of individuals with ASD. Vocational rehabilitation programs are also reviewed in terms of their potential to provide career training and placement for individuals with such disabilities as ASD.

Nonprint Resources

General Autism Resources

Autism Society
http://www.autism-society.org;
Spanish: http://www.autism-society.org/site/
PageServer?pagename=autismo

This is the general Web page for the organization Autism Society that is available in both English and Spanish. The Web site contains general information about autism, ASD-related stories of individuals with ASD and their families, information for professionals, and other important information. Research opportunities as well as treatment options are described in detail. It is a resource for both families and professionals.

Autism Speaks
http://www.autismspeaks.org/

This is the general Web site for the organization Autism Speaks containing a large variety of information, including an introduction to ASD, tools for professionals and families, resources, news about their organized walks, and research initiatives. Many of the tools described in this chapter can be accessed via this home page.

Autism Speaks Family Services Resource Guide and Resource Library
http://www.autismspeaks.org/community/family_services/
tools_for_families.php

In addition to the 100 Day Kit and DVD series, Autism Speaks offers a number of other resources, including state-by-state resources and categories of services available. They do not endorse every resource listed in the guides nor do they claim that the list is comprehensive. The guides are intended to be a starting off point for families seeking services.

Autism Speaks 100 Day Kit
http://www.autismspeaks.org/community/family_services/100_day_kit.php

The Autism Speaks 100 Day Kit is geared toward families whose children have recently been diagnosed with ASD. In addition to containing general information about ASD, it helps families to prioritize the most essential next steps in the 100 days following the diagnosis. It is available free of charge for families with newly diagnosed children under 5 years of age and can be tailored to the individual child depending on his or her age.

First Signs
http://firstsigns.org/

The First Signs organization is dedicated to educating parents, health care providers, early childhood educators, and other professionals about early signs of developmental disorders, including ASD. Their Web site contains information about monitoring childhood development, the screening and referral process, and support for concerns. One of the tools is the ASD Video Glossary, which is also described in this chapter.

Interactive Tools to Track Child Development from the CDC
http://www.cdc.gov/Features/DetectAutismTools/

The Centers for Disease Control and Prevention (CDC) offers interactive tools for parents to help track how a child plays, learns, speaks, and acts. Interactive Milestone Charts and Checklist are offered to teach parents about developmental milestones in order to help recognize when development may be off course. They also offer a video called *Baby Steps: Learn the Signs. Act Early,* which provides information and guidance on identifying developmental disabilities.

Manitas por Autismo, Spanish
http://www.manitasporautismo.com/

This Web site offers information about ASD in Spanish. Available information includes services, general introduction to ASD, and relevant news.

National Institute of Mental Health: Autism
http://www.nimh.nih.gov/health/publications/autism/complete-publication.shtml

National Library of Medicine: Autism
http://www.nlm.nih.gov/medlineplus/autism.html

The National Institute of Mental Health and the National Library of Medicine have compiled a comprehensive information and fact sheets about ASD on their Web sites. Information about etiology, treatment, and resources are included.

OASIS Web site: Online Asperger's Syndrome Information and Support
http://www.udel.edu/bkirby/asperger

Run by the parent of a child with Asperger's, the OASIS Web site has abundant information about Asperger's Disorder for parents, individuals with Asperger's, and professionals. Topics covered include information about the diagnosis and the diagnostic process, support groups, online support, programs (e.g., camps and schools) specific to Asperger's, and information about social skills.

University of Michigan Health Systems
http://www.med.umich.edu/1libr/yourchild/autism.htm

This Web site from the University of Michigan presents information about ASD in a question-and-answer format. In addition to answers to commonly asked questions, it also provides links and ways to obtain further information about related topics. Books and helpful Web sites are also provided.

Films and Video Clips

Adam. 2009. DVD. Directed by Max Meyer.
Santa Monica, CA: Olympus Pictures.
Adam (2009) is a major motion picture about a young man with Asperger's Disorder who becomes romantically involved with a woman living in his apartment complex. It fairly accurately portrays the experience of individuals with Asperger's who are trying to navigate the social world successfully. The movie stars Hugh Dancy and Rose Byrne.

Aging with Autism: Defining the Future. DVDs. 2007.
Commack, NY: Nassau Suffolk Services
for Autism and the Martin C. Barell School.
http://www.autismspeaks.org/community/family_services/
aging_with_autism_dvds.php

Autism Speaks offers the *Aging with Autism: Defining the Future* DVDs free of charge (except for shipping and handling) to parents and professionals interested in learning how to navigate issues that emerge as children with ASD grow older. The DVDs consist of conference proceedings from the *Aging with Autism* conference presented by Developmental Disabilities Institute, Nassau Suffolk Services for Autism, and the Eden II Programs. Autism Speaks recorded many of the sessions to share with families and caregivers who could not attend. Topics included on the series of DVDs include housing and life transitions, sexuality, and employment. This is one of the few resources available specifically for adolescents and adults with ASD.

ASD Video Glossary

http://www.firstsigns.org/asd_video_glossary/asdvg_about.htm

The ASD Video Glossary is a free online resource intended to help parents and professionals become familiar with the early red flags and diagnostic features of ASD. The glossary contains more than a hundred video clips highlighting the, at times, subtle differences between young children who are typically developing and those who have ASD. Clips are categorized by the type of ASD symptom or red flag. The ASD Video Glossary is not intended to help make an ASD diagnosis but rather to show examples of the various types of differences in children with ASD.

Autism Everyday. 2006–2007. DVD Directed by Lauren Thierry. Huntington, NY: Milestone Video.

http://www.autismspeaks.org/sponsoredevents/autism_every_day.php

Autism Everyday is a documentary produced by Eric Solomon and Lauren Thierry in conjunction with Autism Speaks that tells the story and struggles of several families raising their child with autism. It originally premiered in 2006 as a short, 12-minute film and was later expanded in 2007 to 44 minutes. The film is an accurate and powerful portrayal of the day-to-day experience of raising a child with autism.

My Next Steps: A Parent's Guide to Understanding Autism. 2008. DVD. Directed by Raphael Bernier, Jamie Winter, and Jennifer Varley. Seattle, WA: Gigantic Planet.

http://depts.washington.edu/uwautism/video/video.html

My Next Steps: A Parent's Guide to Understanding Autism (2008) is a full-length DVD intended for families who have just received a first-time diagnosis of autism in their child. The DVD is produced by the University of Washington Autism Center and offers guidance to parents through interviews with experts and families. Topics covered include an overview and history of autism, treatment strategies, information about schools, and family stories. DVD chapters can be downloaded at the Web site, and the DVD can be ordered free of charge.

Rain Man. 1988. DVD. Directed by Barry Levinson. Los Angeles, CA: United Artists.

Rain Man (1998) is a film starring Dustin Hoffman and Tom Cruise and was directed by Barry Levinson. Dustin Hoffman provides an accurate portrayal of an adult with autism, Raymond Babbitt, while Tom Cruise plays his long-lost brother. The movie tells the story of the two brothers getting to know each other through a cross-country road trip together. It was the first major motion picture about an individual with autism and was a major contributor to the increasing awareness about autism in the media. The movie won several Academy Awards, including Best Picture.

Environmental Supports: Computer Software, Visual Supports, and Other Materials

Attainment Company
http://www.attainmentcompany.com

The Attainment Company offers many products to help people with disabilities, including ASD, be successful in various aspects of their lives including school, work, and day-to-day living activities. Programs combine pictures, instructional videos, and lesson plans in such products as software to understand money, cook independently, and keep track of their own schedules and time.

Autism Resource Network
http://www.autismshop.com/

This Web site is a relatively comprehensive, one-stop shopping network for materials that may be helpful for families of children with autism. Goods that are sold via the Web site include books, DVDs, visual supports, PECS, and speech/language items including oral motor tools.

Do2Learn
http://www.do2learn.com

Do2Learn is an interactive Web site containing teacher and parent materials that may be helpful for children with ASD. Materials include computer-based instruction, picture cards, and software to make visual schedules. Additionally, the Web site offers a computer program to help children recognize emotions. Special needs resources: http://www.specialneeds.com/.

Laureate Learning Systems
http://www.laureatelearning.com

Laureate Learning Systems offers many computer programs for individual with special needs including ASD, language impairments, developmental disabilities, Down syndrome, aphasia, and traumatic brain injury. Software includes instruction on such areas as cause and effect, vocabulary, syntax, concept development, auditory processing, and reading.

Mayer-Johnson
http://www.mayer-johnson.com

Mayer-Johnson is a company that makes products for individuals with special needs, including ASD, designed to improve communication through such symbols as pictures. It may be helpful for individuals with ASD with limited language and who require alterative ways to communicate.

Social Stories
http://www.thegraycenter.org/

The Gray Center for Social Learning and Understanding was founded by Carol Gray who first defined social stories in 1991. Her social story software is available for purchase on the Web site as well as instructional videos and books. The Web site has further information about social stories and general information about autism.

Visual Strategy Suggestions
http://www.usevisualstrategies.com

Children with autism tend to be better at understanding visual as compared to verbal information. Therefore, they are often described as visual learners and acquire information better with, for example, pictures to accompany verbal information. This Web site is dedicated to providing support, products, and information about visual strategies for children with autism.

Support Resources

Families for Effective Autism Treatment (FEAT), State Chapters
http://www.feat.org/

Families for Effective Autism Treatment (FEAT) is an organization dedicated to informing families about the most current treatment resources available to them. Other supports include respite care, support groups, and recommendations for specific providers. Although there isn't a national Web site, there are Web sites specific to each state or city chapter of FEAT. As an example, the Web site for the northern California chapter (the founding chapter) of FEAT is provided.

MAAP Services for Autism and Asperger Syndrome
http://maapservices.org/

This group is a global information and support network for More Advanced individuals with Autism and Asperger Syndrome, and Pervasive Developmental Disorder (MAAP). MAAP is a nonprofit organization that provides information and advice to families through a quarterly newsletter that be accessed on their Web site. Additional information included on the Web site includes a discussion of families' legal rights, a resource finder, and relevant publications.

Sibling Support Project
http://www.siblingsupport.org/

The Sibling Support Project is a "national effort dedicated to the life-long concerns of brothers and sisters of people who have special health, developmental, or mental health concerns." The project trains local service providers in best practices of providing support to siblings through workshops, Listservs, and peer support programs. "SibShops" are held across the country to fulfill the mission of the Sibling Support Project.

School and Education

Individuals with Disabilities Education Act (IDEA)
http://idea.ed.gov/

IDEA is a federal law that ensures educational services for children with disabilities. This Web site contains information about IDEA for the two different age groups served (birth to 3 years, and 3–21 years). Topics related to evaluation, how IDEA applies to private schools, and the Individual Education Program (IEP), among many other areas, are included.

School Community Toolkit
http://www.autismspeaks.org/community/family_services/school_kit.php

The School Community Toolkit, created by Autism Speaks, is a support for teachers and school staff who interact and work with children with ASD in an educational environment. It is not a specific educational curriculum but rather offers generation information about ASD, overall intervention strategies, and ideas for how to support children with ASD in general education classrooms. The kit can be downloaded for free from the Web site.

Wrightslaw
http://www.wrightslaw.com/

Wrightslaw is a resource page for how the law applies to special education and individuals with disabilities. Books and other resources are available via the Web site as well as articles relating to a variety of relevant topics.

Glossary

Applied Behavioral Analysis (ABA)   ABA is the only intervention approach that research has deemed effective for addressing ASDs. It is a general term that encompasses intervention approaches designed to change behavior. In children with autism, it involves an intensive teaching method of carefully reinforcing certain positive behaviors while decreasing unwanted behaviors. Social and communication skills are usually the focus of ABA. An ABA therapy program is individualized in order to address the child's specific strengths and areas of challenge. It is recommended that ABA begin as early as possible and that therapy should take place for at least 25 hours/week to maximize the effectiveness.

Asperger's Disorder   As with all of the other ASDs, children with Asperger's Disorder (or Asperger's Syndrome) have social difficulties and restricted/repetitive interests. Unlike autism, children with Asperger's do not have a language delay and have average to above-average intelligence as measured by cognitive testing. Asperger's is usually diagnosed later than autistic disorder because children who receive this diagnosis do not have a language delay, so parents are not often concerned as early.

Autism   Autism is also known as "autistic disorder" or "strict autism." Children with a diagnosis of autism struggle in the three areas described under the definition for ASDs. Children with autism generally have a greater number of difficulties than those with diagnosis of Asperger's Disorder or PDD-NOS. Many children with autism also have cognitive disabilities.

Autism Diagnostic Interview (ADI)   The ADI is an assessment tool that is helpful in making a diagnosis of an ASD. It is a 2- to 2.5-hour interview that is done with a child's primary caregiver involving very specific questions about a child's social and language development and sensory and repetitive/restricted behaviors and interests.

Autism Diagnostic Observation Schedule (ADOS)   The ADOS is a well-validated assessment tool that assesses social and communication skills as well as restricted/repetitive interests. It usually lasts 45–60 minutes

297

and consists of 10–14 different play activities designed to elicit social communication.

Autism Spectrum Disorders (ASDs)   ASDs refer to an array of "pervasive developmental disorders." The three main disorders that are included under this umbrella term of ASD are autism, Asperger's Disorder, and PDD-NOS. In general, ASDs are disorders of the brain that begin early in life impacting three basic areas of functioning and development. The first area of functioning is *social* interaction and may include decreased eye contact and minimal back-and-forth social exchanges. The second area of difficulty is *communication* skills (e.g., delayed language and repetitive speech). The final category associated with ASDs is more atypical behaviors including *restricted/repetitive* behaviors and interests, and insistence on routine or sameness. Once considered a rare disorder, the prevalence of ASDs is now increasing in the general population, with current estimates of 1 in 166 children. ASDs are three to four times more common in boys than girls.

Autistic savant   An individual with autism who demonstrates remarkable abilities in a focused area, such as artistic talents or mathematical capabilities. An example might be an individual who can mentally calculate incredibly quickly what day of the week someone's birthday is.

Board-certified behavior analysts (BCBAs)   BCBAs conduct behavioral assessments and provide interpretations of the results of such assessments. They design and supervise behavior analytic interventions to address both the acquisition of skills and the reduction of challenging behaviors. Many BCBAs also hold licenses or certifications in other disciplines (e.g., psychology). These professionals provide behavioral treatments in a variety of locations, but often in the home.

Cognitive testing   Sometimes referred to as "intelligence testing," it is a general term referring to assessments designed to learn more about current verbal and nonverbal problem-solving skills. Cognitive testing includes such activities as making patterns with blocks, completing patterns, and answering questions about words. It is done during many autism evaluations to help determine the best treatment and educational programs for that particular child.

Diagnostic and Statistical Manual of Mental Disorders (DSM)   The *DSM* is a widely used manual that provides a description of all of the specific diagnoses of mental disorders and groups these diagnoses by category. A list of symptoms and diagnostic criteria is specified for all possible diagnoses. Specific codes are assigned to each diagnosis, and providers are able to bill for services provided using these codes. ASDs are under the category of "Pervasive Developmental Disorders." The code for Autistic Disorder is 299.00, Asperger's Disorder is 299.80, and PDD-NOS is 299.80. The *DSM* is currently in its fourth edition, and a fifth edition of the *DSM* is underway in which the sections pertaining to ASDs will be significantly modified.

Echolalia   Echolalia is a term that refers to the repetition of words or phrases heard previously. The echoing can occur immediately after hearing the word or phrase (called immediate echolalia) or can be delayed (called delayed echolalia).

Electroencephalogram (EEG)   A tool that uses electrodes located on the scalp to record electrical activity from the brain. It is used to help aid in the identification of seizures, which many children with autism have.

Facilitated communication (FC)   Facilitated communication is an augmentative communication technique in which an individual selects or points to letters on the keyboard or visual display while a facilitator supports his or her hand, arm, or elbow through the process. Supporters propose that this method allows individuals with autism to communicate effectively, but scientific research suggests that FC is not an effective treatment as it is the facilitators that are communicating *for* the individual with the disability, not the individual with autism.

Individualized Education Program (IEP)   An IEP is a comprehensive document that is designed to make sure that a child with disabilities of any kind (including ASDs) receives appropriate services in a school environment. It includes yearly goals for the child and an intervention plan that it will take to reach those goals. U.S. law requires that every qualified child with a disability have an IEP. Families are involved in the process of developing/updating their child's IEP every school year. Many people (including speech/language pathologists and general/special education teachers) are also involved in meetings to create/update a child's IEP.

Individuals with Disabilities Educational Act (IDEA)   IDEA is a U.S. federal law designed to make sure that children with disabilities have the opportunity to receive a free appropriate public education. IDEA guides how states and school districts provide special education and related services to children with disabilities and early intervention services to infants and toddlers with disabilities. Autism was added as a category of disability eligible for special education services in 1990. The focus of IDEA shifted in 1997 toward an inclusion model, meaning that more importance has been placed on involving children with disabilities into a general education curriculum.

Macrocephaly   Macrocephaly refers to the condition in which an individual's head circumference is two standard deviations over the average—meaning that an individual has a head circumference that is greater than 97 percent of his or her age-matched peers. Many children with autism have macrocephaly.

Magnetic resonance imaging (MRI)   A tool that generates an image of the body, often of the brain. It can be used to aid in the identification of structural abnormalities in the brain. Given that autism is a brain-based disorder, sometimes physicians will request that a child with autism receive an MRI as a follow-up assessment.

Mainstreaming Mainstreaming refers to the placement of a child with disabilities in a regular education classroom with peers with typical development.

Occupational therapy (OT) Therapy provided by an occupational therapist that focuses on the development of sensory, motor, coordination, and self-help skills that aid in daily living. OT is also often recommended for children with a diagnosis of an ASD to address sensory difficulties, fine motor deficits, repetitive motor mannerisms, and daily-living skills.

Perseveration Perseveration refers to the sticking to one idea or action through repetitive movement or speech. Some children with autism are said to *perseverate* on a specific topic of interest, such as toilets or street signs, by talking at length about the topic or extensively focusing attention on the object.

Pervasive Developmental Disorder—Not Otherwise Specified (PDD-NOS) PDD-NOS is often described as "atypical autism" because children with this diagnosis have autism-like features but do not present the same as those with strict autism. For example, children with PDD-NOS may be very interested in social interaction but approach others in a somewhat unusual manner. Additionally, they often have higher language and cognitive skills than those with autistic disorder.

Picture Exchange Communication System (PECS) PECS is a visual support that is intended to help children communicate through the use of pictures in place of verbal language.

Social story A social story is a short, developmentally appropriate story that describes a standard routine (e.g., a trip to the doctor's office) from beginning to end. It also describes any potential difficulties that may be encountered along the way (e.g., "The shot at the doctor might hurt a little, but my mom will be there and it will be alright"). It is designed to help children anticipate future events and to minimize surprises associated with this new event.

Speech-language pathologist A professional who specializes in human communication and provides speech therapy. Speech therapy is often recommended for children who receive a diagnosis of autism because many children with an ASD often have difficulties with language. Speech therapy can focus on improving a child's understanding of language (receptive language), spoken language (expressive language), and conversation skills.

Stereotyped/repetitive interests, language, and motor movements Children with autism often have very specific interests (called "restricted/repetitive interests"), such as in very particular video games, that often take up the majority of the child's time. Stereotyped/repetitive language refers to the tendency for children with autism to repeat certain words/phrases in a very specific way, such as lines from a movie. Stereotyped/repetitive motor movements are repetitive ways of moving the body, such as repeated hand flapping. It may occur more often during stressful situations or periods of excitement.

Stim   A term that is short for "self-stimulation." Self-stimulation refers to behaviors such as repetitive spinning, repetitive movement of the hands or fingers, or other repetitive movements. Many children with autism engage in these types of behaviors. Many propose that these behaviors serve to stimulate one's senses, while others argue the behaviors serve in such self-regulation as calming oneself or shutting out sensory input.

T.E.A.C.C.H. (Treatment and Education of Autism and Related Communication Handicapped Children)   This is an educational treatment approach developed by Eric Schopler based on the idea that many individuals with autism have a relative strength in understanding and using visual cues. Through the use of picture schedules, breaking tasks into steps, and an arranged classroom space, the approach fosters independence.

Theory of mind   Theory of mind is the concept that others have beliefs, desires, and intentions that are different from one's own. Many scientists suggest that individuals with autism have deficits in theory of mind.

Visual schedule   A visual schedule is a method of providing a schedule for the day in pictures. Given that many children with autism have a relative strength in using and understanding visual cues but also struggle with transitions, this is a technique that is sometimes used to aid in maximizing understanding of a schedule.

Index

About the Authors

DR. RAPHAEL BERNIER is a licensed clinical psychologist and a faculty member at the University of Washington in the Department of Psychiatry and Behavioral Sciences and adjunct faculty member in the Department of Psychology. Dr. Bernier's research focuses on the etiology, neuroscience, and behavioral presentation of Autism Spectrum Disorders and childhood disorders. Dr. Bernier holds an undergraduate degree from Tufts University, a graduate degree from the University of Wisconsin–Madison, and a PhD from the University of Washington.

JENNIFER GERDTS, MS, is a graduate student in the Department of Psychology, Child Clinical program at the University of Washington. She has worked at the University of Washington Autism Center on a variety of research projects and provided various clinical services to families. Her research focus is in the behavioral presentation of Autism Spectrum Disorders and the patterns of autism-related traits in families. Gerdts obtained her undergraduate degree in psychology from Colby College and her MS in child clinical psychology at the University of Washington. She will receive her PhD in 2012.